FAT, BROKE
& LONELY
No More!

Also by Victoria Moran:

Creating a Charmed Life:
Sensible, Spiritual Secrets Every Busy Woman Should Know

Fit from Within:
101 Simple Secrets to Change Your Body and Your Life

Lit from Within:
A Simple Guide to the Art of Inner Beauty

Shelter for the Spirit:
Create Your Own Haven in a Hectic World

Younger by the Day:
365 Ways to Rejuvenate Your Body and Revitalize Your Spirit

FAT, BROKE & LONELY
No More!

Your Personal Solution to
Overeating, Overspending, and
Looking for Love in All the Wrong Places

VICTORIA MORAN

HarperOne
A Division of HarperCollinsPublishers

HarperOne

FIRST EDITION

Designed by Joseph Rutt

Library of Congress Cataloging-in-Publication Data is available upon request.

ISBN: 978-0-06-115423-2
ISBN-10: 0-06-115423-7

07 08 09 10 11 RRD(H) 10 9 8 7 6 5 4 3 2 1

With love and appreciation to my two mothers—

Dede, my first spiritual teacher and real-life "Auntie Mame":
You gave me magic and wonder.
I'm doing my best to pass those on.

And Mom, with all your spunk and your irrepressible spirit:
You were so with me as I wrote this book,
I know we did it together.

CONTENTS

Part Two

BREAKING UP WITH FAT

*There is a power inside you that leads to right decisions,
even in areas as ordinary as your food choices
and getting to the gym.*

Part Three

BREAKING UP WITH BROKE

*Abundance—financial and otherwise—is normal, natural, and right.
You attract it by thinking, speaking, and living abundantly.*

Part Four

BREAKING UP WITH LONELY

*When your life is full and your spirit engaged,
you'll delight in your own company and draw caring,
supportive people into your world.*

Part Five

HOOKING UP WITH THE LIFE OF YOUR DREAMS

You came to this planet to be remarkable.
You do that by being yourself, using your gifts,
and shining your light.

INTRODUCTION

As the reader of this book, you deserve to be in on how it came about. My editor called and said, "We've been playing with a title we really like, but we didn't know who could write it. Then it occurred to me: *you* could write it!" I loved that he'd thought of me to take on this title, surely something graceful and gracious, beautiful and uplifting. "'*Fat, Broke & Lonely*'!" he announced enthusiastically. I felt as if I'd been punched.

You see, I've *been* fat, broke & lonely, and I don't like these words—especially *fat*, because I was hurt the most by that one. I haven't been overweight in more than twenty years, but I am still well aware that *fat* isn't a mere synonym for *overweight*. In our society, *fat* is a somatic epithet, a judgment, and a weapon. To this day, when I know that someone else has been stung by the word, I flinch with that person. *Broke* and *lonely* are less piercing but scarcely more appealing. The three words together paint a picture no one wants to see. Nevertheless, before I could say, "I wouldn't write a book called that in a million years," I remembered something: although I have been fat, broke & lonely, I'm not anymore, and I haven't been for some time.

This is how I see it today: there is shared culpability for the problem. We are responsible for our actions, but "they" aren't making it any easier. *They* include the giant corporations that produce much of our food and the planning commissions that decide to build developments without sidewalks. *They* are the advertisers who adroitly convince us that we ought to be able to buy everything they're peddling and still come up with the money for the next status symbol or must-have toy. And living in a society short on the extended families and close communities that human beings have depended on since before we first walked upright is undeniably one of the reasons so many of us feel lonely and disconnected.

You deserve to take a minute (or as long as you need) to feel righteously outraged at a culture that makes it so easy to be fat, broke & lonely. When you're finished, though, it's still up to you to find a way out.

As someone who's done that, I figured my editor had a point: I'm supposed to share what I know with people who want it. This includes individuals who might describe themselves as fat and/or broke and/or lonely, and the many others who are just so afraid of ending up there that they run themselves ragged at the gym, on the job, and in their relationships. They're operating under the logical assumption that a *perfect* person couldn't possibly be fat, broke & lonely, so doing everything perfectly has to be the best cover. But after the killer workout, the plum assignment, and the dream date, the fear of becoming fat, broke & lonely hasn't gone anywhere.

Obviously, I said I'd write the book. We tweaked the title to *Fat, Broke & Lonely No More*. Being able to say, "No more!" in your own life—and mean it—has less to do with food or money or the people who are (or are not) sending you text-messages than it does with you, on the inside. Your core beliefs. What you want for yourself. Your spirituality.

Don't blow this off as New Age mumbo-jumbo or the sole purview of the baptized, born again, or bat-mitzvahed. I'm simply urging you to understand that there is more going on than our five senses can fathom, that you're more remarkable than you may have realized, and that you have some control, via your thoughts, words, and attitude, over how you experience life. For example, when you focus on fat, broke & lonely, that's what shows up: "I'm fat and disgusting—I need to eat something.... I'll never have enough money—I need to buy something.... I'll never meet the right person—I need to call what's-his-name. I mean, he only had that one DUI and something could have been wrong with the Breathalyzer...."

I wrote *Fat, Broke & Lonely No More* to help you part company with this plague once and for all. For this to work, you'll have to put what you read here into practice. Every chapter ends with the directive "Take an action." Your actions, far more than my words, will make the difference. Your actions will give you access to the missing ingredient that, like caulk or Hamburger Helper, can fill the empty places. With it, there's always enough, and this sufficiency feels like a banquet. Or a trust fund. Or a standing ovation.

Part One

BREAKING UP WITH THE EMPTINESS INSIDE

Fat, broke & lonely arises from an inner void and withdraws when you develop a viable inner life.

Although abetted by culture and commerce, fat, broke & lonely is essentially a response to an emptiness inside. If you could break it off with fat, broke & lonely by merely eating less, working harder, and being friendly, you'd have done it. So would everybody else. It's not that simple. Remember: fat, broke & lonely looks like a straightforward description of a state of being, but it's really a way people are controlled through shame and fear. Discovering and nurturing your inner self is essential for seeing through the lies that fat, broke & lonely tells to the truth of who you are: a being of purpose and power, a person with a reason to be here and important work to do.

The ten chapters that follow will give you tools to develop and deepen the inner part of yourself. This is where the strength will come from to keep you secure in where you are and out of the reach of fat, broke & lonely—and anything else that might want to interfere with your living an incredible life.

Chapter 1

THE ANATOMY OF
FAT, BROKE & LONELY

Fat, broke & lonely. These words haven't routinely been grouped together like backup singers, and yet this trio represents the overarching personal fear of our era. Of course we're concerned about terrorist attacks and melting polar ice caps, but we can feel so powerless over those that there's no use obsessing about them. Fat, broke & lonely, however, can take front and center. We either give in to it by overeating, overspending, and looking for love in all the wrong places, or confront it with steely resolve: "No matter what else happens, by golly, I can look great, have the right stuff, and know the right people."

Not that there's anything wrong with wanting these. In evolutionary terms, they're inextricably linked to our primal instincts to survive and procreate. When wanting turns to craving, however, that desperation posts an open invitation to fat, broke & lonely.

In my observations, women seem to be the most apprehensive about being either fat or lonely. In many women's minds, these are two sides of the same coin. Being fat (or unattractive—a pimple or bad blow-dry can feel like three pounds around the midsection) carries with it the threat of not being loved romantically or even liked platonically. And if loneliness comes first, fat may well follow. When there's a breakup on a sitcom, for example, the gal is going to be eating ice cream out of the carton before the next commercial.

For men, *broke* is often a bogeyman more heinous than fat and lonely combined. Although men are increasingly being pressured to succumb to the same impossible body-beautiful messages that bombard women, fat need not be fatal to the masculine self-image as long as the man is successful, powerful, and well-to-do. The pain of loneliness is not gender-specific, but men have been socialized for self-reliance, and most cultures have long allowed single men the comfort of casual encounters while frowning upon them for women. A man lacking means, however, feels impotent to attract females, impress males, and fulfill his evolutionary mandate to support a family (even when his wife's income could support the family, and perhaps then he feels it even more).

Individual interpretations and gender divides notwithstanding, each of these words is loaded. Whatever truth they're supposed to convey is overshadowed by the half-truths, inferences, and bold-faced lies they also communicate. Certainly there's the "fat" that's a health risk, and then there's "Do I look fat in these jeans?" asked to elicit the response, "Are you kidding? You're so skinny, you look gorgeous in everything."

Broke, too, doesn't usually mean "penniless." I was shocked to hear my husband lament early in our marriage (second time for both—we weren't kids), "We're so broke I don't eat lunch!" We were earning six figures, and in cooperation with the bank, we owned an imposing stone house from the Arts and Crafts era. The extensive (and expensive) work required to rehab it, though, caused William to regard a sandwich as a luxury and *broke* as an applicable adjective.

Similarly, *lonely* usually doesn't mean "all alone." We define it as "without a life partner" (or with the wrong one), or as lacking in the number or type of friends or social contacts we think we should have or believe we once did. "I had so many friends in college [or when I lived in Minneapolis, or before I was on the road so much], but I just can't connect with people now."

Taken in tandem, though, fat, broke & lonely isn't shorthand for having some weight to lose, being low on cash this month, and requesting a table for one the second night in a row. At its root, fat, broke & lonely, whether as fact or fear, arises from emptiness inside a human being, a cavity in the soul. Eating too much food (or worrying too much about eating food), spending too much money (or expecting too much from money), and depending too much on others (or pushing them away) all stem from a void at the core. This book could have been called *Drunk, Bummed & Worried No More,* or *Frustrated, Exhausted & Dissed No More,* or *Starving Myself, Scared to Death & Sleeping Around No More.* Any of these (without the "no more") can rob us of the best stuff: the present moment, our next brilliant idea, the people who think we're fabulous.

The key to breaking up with fat, broke & lonely is the realization that *you really are enough,* that you can feel full on the inside because nothing is lacking. This is what it takes to feel nourished (and beautiful), prosperous (and safe), loved (and loving), and, in the rock-solid here and now, to eat well and get fitter, earn more and invest wisely, and attract people into your life who'll be there for you no matter what.

To dump fat, broke & lonely, you're going to have to meet your inner emptiness head-on and deal with it. But before you add another agony to the list ("Oh, my God, I'm fat, broke, lonely, and empty too!"), be advised: it's not just you. That is to say, you're not troubled about how you look, how much you have, and who you're with because you have some *condition*. (I'm astounded that virtually every human challenge is now a condition that can be treated with a really remarkable drug—if you don't mind side effects like intermittent spleen pain, rampant growth of back hair, and herpes of the eye.) This whole fat-broke-and-lonely thing isn't just you, it's also your culture, one that has a vested interest in keeping you troubled about your shortcomings, real and imagined.

You're needed to support both the doughnut and diet-food industries. You're expected to say yes to the credit cards, with their irresistible introductory rates, and to fill a seat at the make-a-mint-in-real-estate seminar. The status quo depends on your purchasing the latest styles and newest cosmetics, which will cause men to lust after you and women to admire you and seek out your company.

Good grief, if you and I and everyone we know weren't so busy dealing with fat, broke & lonely, we could be ending starvation, curing AIDS, and making "peace on earth" something more than a message on a Christmas card. We could even have fun for the sake of having fun and not because it's burning calories or helping us network.

The way to get from here to there is by getting in touch on a regular basis with the wisdom inside you that, when you've listened to it, has been known to impart inklings that impressed the heck out of you. This clarifying and connecting balances your various needs and drives and instincts and puts them in perspective. It gives you autonomy, so that what you're told you're supposed to be has no authority over who you know you are. Your waist measurement, bank balance, and plans for Saturday night no longer define you, and you know that the power to change any of them resides within you. It's been there all along, and it's not going anywhere.

Take an Action

Notice every time fat, broke & lonely affects your life today. How often do you think about one or more of these conditions? Worry about them? Put yourself down in relation to them? Think less of another person in relation to them? Envy another person who seems invulnerable to them?

Chapter 2

THE EMPTINESS EPIDEMIC

When Peggy Lee sang "Is That All There Is?" her response to feeling empty inside was "Let's keep dancing." Most of us, however, react to that sense of not having, doing, or being *enough* with filler behaviors that are far more insidious than tripping the light fantastic. Eating, spending, and isolating—among the building blocks of fat, broke & lonely—are favorites. Overdrinking (Ms. Lee's song went on to suggest "break[ing] out the booze"), overworking, and even overgiving show up too. So do worry, anger, and fear, as well as changing jobs, addresses, or love interests, but none of these works very well or for very long.

The information age exists simultaneously with an emptiness epidemic that statistics bear out: 62 percent of American adults are overweight, including the 31 percent who are obese. (The flip side of fatness, anorexia, is a growing problem as well, and it now affects boys, men, and middle-aged women as well as the adolescent girls who once cornered the market on self-starvation.) Until recent legislation made bankruptcy more difficult, 100,000 Americans were filing every month, suggesting that a lot of folks are, despite the plastic in their pockets, broke. With 52 percent of marriages ending in divorce, 85 million empty-nesters, and the rest of us yakking about the dysfunctional families we can't stand to be around, loneliness is rampant as well. And the dread of these makes almost everybody *feel* fat, broke & lonely at times, or at least in imminent danger of fitting one of these descriptions.

Fear has created fact. We're told to strive for thinness, success, and admiration in order to justify our very existence, but our desperation to achieve or maintain these brings on their antithesis. Everybody knows about the dance of the diet and the binge: if you diet severely, you lose weight, but you gain it back at lightning speed because the body's need to maintain homeostasis, balance, steps in to attempt to bring things back to normal. (Of course, when obese people are tortured into slimness on TV, we applaud the biggest loser, even though mountains of evidence tell us that dropping weight quickly comes with a virtual guarantee of regaining it and more.)

When it comes to money, we're supposed to have plenty of it, and if we don't, we need to appear as if we do. Going into the red for the right clothes in which to be seen with the right people at the right places is purportedly an investment in the future, even when it's putting us deeper in the hole. Loneliness escalates as we seek out friends and partners based on how they look, how much they have, and what they can do for us. When they're not around, there are people we can watch on TV, those we can "chat" with in cyberspace, and the ones who serenade us through our headsets. Most of us "know" far more people than know us back—a historically recent phenomenon to which our emotional natures have not had the time to adapt.

In the emptiness epidemic, we're prisoners of extremes. Outside of fat liberation circles, you'd be hard-pressed to find a person in this culture who wants to be obese. The problem arises when media messages imply that anyone carrying around more than 19 percent body fat has entered the zone of the unredeemed. You're supposed to work tirelessly to rid yourself of this blight, worry about it the rest of the time, and understand that until your body passes muster, you do not deserve a full and fulfilling life.

It's not so different with money and social acceptance. Except in religious sects that prize poverty, nobody wants to be broke. But is society celebrating the woman who paid off her student loans and credit card debt, lives proudly on a cash basis, and is tucking away a portion of every paycheck? Hardly. We're too busy looking up to heiresses and moguls with busy PR firms. And other than the occasional wandering ascetic, the contented recluse, and Greta Garbo, nobody signs on for a friendless existence. But again, we're handed a nearly unachievable ideal: becoming the perfect man or woman (hot body, fat bank account, on every A-lister's A-list) with a host of perfect friends (although some of them can be a little less perfect than you so you'll look better).

You're given impossible goals coupled with the message that if you fall short even a little, you'll be relegated to fat, broke & lonely, and there's nothing worse than that. Probably the most basic tenet of metaphysics, however, is this: *what you focus on, you attract.* This tells me that staying out of the reach of fat, broke & lonely is achieved by getting involved with their legitimate opposites: healthy fitness, financial well-being, and satisfying relationships. The opposites of fat, broke & lonely according to the media, however, are impossible thinness, incredible wealth, and the admiration of the multitudes.

A part of you knows that you can't focus on such a flimsy fantasy, so your attention goes the only place it can—to fat, broke & lonely. This diligent visualization, even when unconscious, either brings the three horsemen of emptiness galloping into your experience or keeps you stuck in the dread of them. Here's the paradox: when you let go of the belief that fat, broke & lonely is the worst fate that can befall a person, you'll be trimmer, richer, and happier.

This is a major leap because we're talking about fundamental issues: the way you appear to yourself and others, your health, your financial security, your sex life, and your family, friends, and future. The suggestion I'm making—to get a handle on the underlying emptiness instead of wrestling with its symptoms—can be terrifying. "Good grief! If I'm this fat dieting, I'd be a blimp if I stopped," you may think, or, "My biological clock is going nuts: I have to go out with every guy who asks me." It also takes a lot of work to shut out the print and electronic images of people who were either born resistant to fat, broke & lonely, or who put forth effort so precise and unwavering that they burst through the fat-broke-&-lonely barrier to become one of the anointed, worthy of worship and emulation.

But know this: every human being comes equipped with *essential emptiness*. In the seventeenth century, Blaise Pascal wrote, "There is a God-shaped hole in every man that only God can fill." If you don't like the word *God* (or the word *man* for that matter), use a different word (there's a whole list of deific synonyms in chapter 8), but you get the idea. This essential emptiness is implanted in every human being to cause us to search for meaning. The *epidemic emptiness* affecting so many of us now is an exaggeration and perversion of essential emptiness. It's the difference between feeling hungry because it's time to eat, and a midmorning compulsion to scarf down two bags of chips and a pastry chaser.

Here at the outset, you have a dual assignment. The first is to make peace with essential emptiness and let it spur you to wonderful things—asking questions, contemplating big ideas, and reading this book and lots of others as you search for clues about what's important and satisfying and true. The second part of your assignment is to make peace with the emptiness epidemic: it's not going away, and unless you move to a deserted island, you'll see evidence of it every day. Even on your deserted island, the epidemic could wash ashore when the cast and crew of some reality show decides to shoot there. The idea is to live in the midst of the epidemic but develop immunity to its more disabling aspects.

You can start by recognizing the difference between your natural longing for a more fulfilling life (essential emptiness) and the tormenting craving for something to fill you up right this minute. Your thing might be ravishing the hors d'oeuvres or downing the cocktails, spending every cent or hoarding it away, needing sex on the first date (or as the first date), or being employee of the month yet again because once is never enough. Your role here is not to judge yourself or even stop yourself. Just notice. When you see yourself doing something that leaves you emptier than before, you've observed evidence of the epidemic in a single human life—your own. Not to worry: it isn't fatal. You're collecting information. You are, in fact, gathering truth—and that's the stuff that sets you free.

Take an Action

Make a list of every good thing, major and minuscule, that makes you feel full. A sample list might start: seeing my best friend, being with my children, hearing live music, going to dance class, reading anything Jane Austen wrote. When you have your list, pick one item and do it by this time tomorrow.

Chapter 3

TO GO WHERE OTHER PEOPLE ONLY DREAM OF, DO WHAT THEY WON'T DO

If you could MapQuest fat, broke & lonely, it would say, "Take Easy Street as far as it goes." That's because fat, broke & lonely is the termination of the path of least resistance.

One evening my husband and I were having dinner at a neighborhood trattoria in New York City. We were seated by the window with only a pane of glass between us and the sidewalk. Among the diverse passersby was a man, apparently destitute and undoubtedly drunk. In fact, he could barely stagger, and at one point a fellow walker lurched to grab him before he stumbled into traffic.

I thought about that lost soul for a long time after. He was living at one extreme. At the other are the people we admire: the athlete who breaks records in her youth and breaks barriers for others later on; the scientist who discovers something

important and useful; the once-in-a-blue-moon world leader
whose integrity and insights leave his country and everybody
else's freer and more secure.

In between is everybody else. Some people are struggling
to survive; others are striving to make a difference. There's no
question that luck and circumstance have a role, and in some
cases a substantial one, but once you've taken those into account, willingness, perseverance, and self-control are the factors in play. With these, the man I saw that evening could
most likely have sobered up, gotten a job, and made a positive contribution. Thousands before him have, and they also
make the best motivational speakers you'd ever want to hear.
On the other hand, people at the top of their game can slip to
the bottom with one shady business deal or unwise sexual
encounter. Just staying where you are takes some effort.
Rising above it takes a lot.

We're not instinctually equipped to *want* to get up when
the sun does, meditate or write in a journal, go for a run, fix a
healthy breakfast, and still leave for work early enough to
avoid what-if-I'm-late stress. Few people *want* to go the extra
mile, let someone else be right, learn an intimidating computer program, ask for a raise. After an exhausting day, nobody's natural instincts would choose cleanse, tone, and
moisturize, a little yoga, and flossing over hitting the sack
without the preliminaries. But life belongs to those who floss.

Sure, we're all fond of ease and comfort. When you desire
them more than you desire a quality life, however, you end up
in bed with fat, broke & lonely. The people we think of as extraordinary are usually no smarter or better positioned or
luckier than a whole lot of other people. They are, however,

more disciplined. While those around them are doing the minimum required to maintain the existing state of affairs, men and women with extraordinary lives do a great deal more—when they feel like it and when they don't, consistently, day in, day out.

The rest of us go in fits and starts. We get on a "gym kick," or we go through a "culture phase." After a while, appealing memories of the status quo lure us back to the recliner and the reruns. The key to living in a way that fat, broke & lonely can't touch is to get back in the game as soon as you realize you're out of it. This doesn't come from kicks and phases. It arises from inserting, one at a time, features of the life you want into the life you've got. When you see that you've fallen into an old pattern, get back to the new one. Otherwise, you'll be caught up in a soap opera with only one plot.

Be aware that you and I and anyone with a propensity toward fat, broke & lonely have a compendium of excuses thicker than the Yellow Pages. "I'm tired.... I don't feel good.... It's raining.... She hurt my feelings.... Nobody will know.... It's not that important.... I can start over tomorrow.... It's not my job.... The dog ate my homework...." Well, maybe we haven't used that last one in a while, but you get my point. What's diabolical about excuses is that they look as if they're our allies, helping us out, easing our burdens, when in fact they're creating burdens—fat, broke & lonely among them. Watch for the excuses you routinely use to talk yourself into doing what you know you'd be better off not doing, and the ones that jump in to cover for not doing the tedious, rigorous, humbling, or bothersome task at hand.

A while back a friend told me that she'd read about a new psychiatric disorder. It was some grouping of initials that wasn't ADD or ADHD or any of the ones I'd heard of. These initials, she told me, stood for "knowing what you ought to do but doing something else." I thought the letters for that were B-E-I-N-G H-U-M-A-N. I told her so, and backed up my position with a two-thousand-year-old confession from St. Paul, who wrote, "That which I would do I do not, and that which I would not do I do daily." Her conclusion: "He must have had it too."

However you see it and however you spell it, we like what's easy and we dislike what isn't. Nevertheless, having a shot at the life you're after is going to take doing what you have to do, whether you like it or not. You may choose to do more thinking about all this, read more books, get more counseling, and that's your business, but to ditch fat, broke & lonely sooner rather than later, action trumps analysis every time.

Everybody is a creature of habit. Even my cat gets up at 6:00 A.M. (my alarm clock is a meow), expects some ritual nose-touching (it's a cat thing), and then dashes to the kitchen for breakfast. It's always at that time, always in that order. The almost universal penchant for routine is what makes bad habits so hard to break, but we can use it to turn new ways of being into habits as well. Start with one that's reasonably easy—eating breakfast if you haven't been, looking up unfamiliar words you come upon when you're reading, or clearing off your desk at the end of the day. Do this one simple thing for a month to allow the new pattern to begin to become a part of you. It doesn't mean you're home free: the old way will seem "normal" for a lot longer than thirty days. But it's a start. Your vigilance will make it permanent.

Self-doubt is the greatest enemy of any new good habit. Should your opinion of yourself plummet one day to such a low level that you no longer feel worthy of having a bowl of cereal or finding out what *trenchant* means, you won't do it. You don't give up on what you need to be doing because you are lazy or stupid or destined to be fat, broke & lonely. *You give up on what you need to be doing because you forget that you're worth it.*

This is why most people aren't leading exemplary lives. This is why fat, broke & lonely is less the exception than the rule. You have to believe in yourself so much that you're willing to do what's uncomfortable, time-consuming, inconvenient, and on occasion seemingly impossible. When you don't believe in yourself this much, pretend. You do deserve a great body, a great job, and a great relationship. During a period when you don't have one of these, revel in the others and live so well that the missing element can't help but rush in to complete the picture.

If it's hard for you to feel so entitled, take a lesson from the ruling class. Should that sound like a phrase from the history books, wake up and smell the Dom Pérignon: the ruling class is still here and, to a great extent, still ruling. I'm not suggesting that these people are paragons of mental health—in some cases, far from it—but they were given certain tools early on that can serve the rest of us well too.

Key in the formation of an individual in this demographic is the concept of privilege, of having the right to certain expectations. We all have that right—we just have to learn to exercise it. Educational philosopher John Taylor Gatto has done extensive research on the curricula of the elite private boarding schools along the Eastern Seaboard. These are the institutions that "prep" students not just for Ivy League universities but for positions of power in business, politics, and diplomacy. While public schools seek to give students the tools to become good citizens and competent workers or professionals, the top private schools train their students to wield power. "Access is a major emphasis in these schools, access to whatever aspect of society the individual wishes to join," says Gatto. "The rest of us were taught to memorize the dots but never, never to connect them."

You may not aspire to run a corporation or a country, but you need to connect enough dots to put you in a position of power over fat, broke & lonely. This isn't a matter of feeling that you're better or more deserving than the next person, but rather of knowing that you're good enough and fully deserving simply because you *are* a person. Besides, being entitled doesn't mean having everything handed to you on a platter, silver or otherwise. It means that you're entitled to do the work that will keep you from falling prey to fat, broke & lonely, and that work just might bring you face-to-face with the life you've been meant to discover all along.

Take an Action

Eleanor Roosevelt said, "Do the thing you know you cannot do." That's today's action. What seems difficult or even impossible? Making it through an entire day without criticizing one single person, even under your breath or inside your head? Starting your memoir, even though somebody told you that since you're not famous nobody cares? Splitting from the wrong guy and not even looking for the right one until you've had some time to get to know your glorious self? Today stop debating and leap. Am I asking you to perform an extraordinary feat? You bet I am. But once you've done it, you can do anything.

Chapter 4

GET BUSY ON YOUR MISSION ALREADY

Everybody's busy. The only time I hear the word *bored* these days is from a cohort at the health club who's putting in forty minutes on the treadmill. Nearly everyone else complains about being "exhausted," "overwhelmed," "burned out." This kind of depletion can come from juggling too many balls and wearing too many hats. It can arise from trying to *do* enough in order to feel that you *are* enough, when in fact doing, as vital as it is, is never going to equal being, no matter how diligent your efforts. A great deal of the used-up, caught-in-a-trap, how-did-I-get-into-this way of being results from doing everything on earth except what brought you to earth: your mission.

You do have one. It's imprinted on your soul like a stamp on a passport. Although it may take some time to figure out what your mission is, once you do you can work at it with all that's in you and wake up the next day eager to start again. When you're engaged in your right work, whether for pay or for passion, there's a continual sense of newness about it. An excitement. You came equipped with the aptitudes to take on your mission, and when you do you'll find that you're also equipped with the energy required to go the distance. In addition, you'll realize that you have a direct line to insights regarding this work that you haven't had with other pursuits.

If you don't know what your mission is, that's okay. Most people don't. Now that you know you have one, you can start to discover it. Ask yourself: what did I want to do with my life when I was a little kid (under seven years old if you can think back that far)? Anthroposophist Rudolph Steiner originated a theory of child development that until age seven, or when the permanent teeth begin to come in, a child can be seen as having one foot on earth and the other still in heaven. The newly minted human thrives on imagination and the natural world, fairy tales and fantasy. If you can think back to the way you saw yourself then and remember the sort of person you felt yourself to be, it will help you get in touch with your mission, your calling.

What did you love to do when you were little? Were you drawing or putting on shows or raising a brood of doll children? Were you building cardboard cities, bringing home strays, or playing dress-up every chance you got? Even though you've since acquired education, experience, and sufficient nutrition to grow up, this amazing child, this being fresh from the stars, is still who you are. That mission you sensed when you were too young to name it is the one still inside you.

You can learn more about your mission by looking at where your unique life energy goes when it's not interfered with. Answer these questions, preferably in writing:

- What places feel so good to you that you could stay there forever? Catalog as many as you can think of. Although they can be as diverse as "the beach in Jamaica" and "the downtown library," look for their subtle similarities.

- What sort of movies do you like? What TV programs do you never miss? What kind of book can you not put down? What is the common thread here?

- Who are the people you most enjoy being with? Is there a single quality that all of them share?

- What gives you that wonderful sense of uplift, a lightness that makes you feel as if you could fly?

- Whose sadness and suffering affects you most—that of children, animals, the poor and disenfranchised, the old, the sick?

- If you could be doing anything at this moment, what would it be?

- If there were no limitations of funding, staff, or connections, if you weren't too old, too young, too inexperienced, or too whatever, what would you be engaged in as your life's work?

- If you could change just one thing on this planet for the better, what would it be?

- When you think of the phrase "to make one's mark," what mark do you want to leave?

Your answers to these questions, along with your memory of your childhood self, will provide clues to your mission. I suggest that you take these queries seriously and that you write out answers to each of them with a pen instead of a computer. Writing on paper is a way to gain access to deeper parts of yourself than you can reach with cursory keyboarding.

In addition, look to people who are already involved with their mission. These can be people you know personally and those you've read about. History is filled with big-time mission people, and your local newspaper will tell you of men and women who are on a mission now, right where you live. There's the woman working to get teenage prostitutes off the streets, the entrepreneurial couple who defied the giants and run a successful independent business, the retirees who maintain a garden sanctuary in the center of town.

Getting busy on your mission does not necessarily mean that you'll show up in the history books or the papers. In fact, in this era of uncensored show-and-tell, there is something incredibly classy about remaining anonymous, quietly changing some bit of this planet without media coverage and awards ceremonies. A lovely way to negotiate the public-private balance of your mission is to keep personal glory out of the picture as much as you can. If your mission requires shouting from the housetops (or proffering sound bites on TV), shout or schmooze as necessary. You'll empower your mission by focusing more on its aim than on how terrific you look in blue, but, gosh, if you can do good and look good at the same time, fantastic.

Besides, even a mission that is small in scale can be huge in impact, because once you bring your mission into being, other people get to be a part of it. I felt this when I had the opportunity to speak at Sundance, Robert Redford's mountain retreat in Utah. Originally a home in the country for the actor and his family, Sundance now also enables its many visitors to live harmoniously with nature and do creative work in an inspiring setting. When I was there, luxuriating in the beauty of the place, I thought about how, as a kid, I used to wonder why my mom or my friend couldn't remember their part in the dream I'd had the night before. At Sundance I felt that I'd been allowed inside Robert Redford's dream—not a sleeping dream, but the other kind, a vision. When you bring your mission into being, you give shape and form to a vision that other people can visit, contribute to, and benefit by.

You can certainly have more than one mission in a life. Raising children is a mission of the loftiest order. People who live fulfilled lives all the way through, however, go on to discover a further mission after their kids are launched. Sometimes one mission feeds the next. My first literary agent, for instance, spent her professional life seeing that helpful books made their way into the world. This work enabled her to retire in her forties and become a full-time activist and philanthropist. Like any growing thing, your mission isn't a static entity. It's a work in progress, evolving all the time.

When you're involved in your mission—or even in actively looking for what it might be—you're on fire. The selfish concerns that exist for all of us graciously abate while you're immersed in your calling. In this state, you don't need anything except to keep at it. Then there's nowhere to be but in the moment, and no way to feel but complete.

Take an Action

Answer in writing the questions asked in this chapter. Expect your mission to be revealed to you, along with ways to bring it into being. Be patient. Your mission isn't a project to check off your list. It's a commitment to which to dedicate your life.

Chapter 5

IT DOESN'T MATTER WHAT YOU DO FOR YOUR LIVING: YOUR *LIFE* IS SUPPOSED TO BE ART

Life is tough for artists, especially in the United States, where we celebrate stars and don't seem to care much if the equally talented but undiscovered juggle three jobs and have to clean their voice teacher's apartment in exchange for lessons. When I was looking for a part-time administrative assistant, I put an ad on craigslist and got over two hundred responses in a weekend. The majority of applicants were artists—painters, filmmakers, actors, dancers, writers, musicians. They had BFAs and MFAs. Some had earned honors at Barnard and Brown and NYU. Their plays had been produced, their photographs hung in galleries, and still they were looking for a way to earn a little money with a "B" job (it's not art, but it's okay) or a "C" job (it's close to intolerable, but the rent is due).

To someone looking in from the outside, clinging to one's art despite the hardships it can cause doesn't look all that different from staying in an impossible relationship and hoping something will change when nothing ever has before. But it's not the same. Art can be energizing down to the roots of your being. It puts you on intimate terms with beauty when there's ugliness all around. During the creative process, you get face time with your Higher Self even if you didn't meditate that morning (although meditation—see chapter 9—fuels creativity the way complex carbs fuel a long-distance run). Artists tend to stay with their art through good times and bad because in their sculpting or singing or whatever they do, they are more alive than ever.

My mom used to make a coconut-and-booze confection she called "Better Than Sex Cake." Art is like that: better than sex or chocolate or winning the lottery because it's sustaining, it's self-contained, and it never makes you feel fat or leaves you wondering if he'll call.

It is a fact that lots of artists use alcohol, drugs, sex, food, and money in destructive ways, but that's because many artists, like many non-artists, haven't made the connection between art and life. The lightbulb hasn't gone on in their heads that the lifeblood of creativity—and the secret to wresting every soupçon of satisfaction out of life—is making a work of art out of each and every day.

True creative geniuses are those who understand that a stage or a paintbrush is not required for making the highest art of all. Their medium is the twenty-four-hour period, and their lives are their masterpieces. They're the ones who use the company dishes when there's no company. They put plaid with stripes or green with lavender in a way that works. They buy fresh flowers even if paying for them means they'll have to hand-wash the blouse they'd otherwise have sent to the dry cleaners. "Real artists know they can slice themselves every which way," says Necia Gamby, a mentor of mine and an elder (i.e., my age) visionary in the hip-hop community. "The most important thing to an artist is having a way to express, no matter which channel of expression you're looking at."

Similarly, you'll feel filled (and fulfilled) when your life overall is a work of art. This is not about perfectionism— making sure you never kick back, take time off, get dirty, make mistakes, or hang up your halo. Life-as-art is above all else *interesting*. It's textured, intriguing, unique, and worth taking a look at. As with a film or a song, your life-as-art is not going to be appreciated by everyone. Some people (certain relatives probably, and envious peers) will heartily disapprove. That's the risk every artist takes. When a painter or a poet tones down his work simply to gain a wider audience, we say he has sold out. You and I sell out, too, when we color our lives neatly inside the lines.

Live creatively if you don't already, and if you do, do it some more. See your day as a canvas to paint or a lump of clay to mold into something beautiful and useful. To get started, answer these artsy questions:

- What do you use to wash your face? Is it just some product you picked up somewhere, or did you think before you bought it about how it feels and smells and works with your complexion? Was it tested on animals?

Are the ingredients as safe and natural as those you look for in your food?

- What about your toothpaste? Is it the same old mint stuff your mother bought for you, or have you discovered imported, specialty, *artistic* toothpastes?

- When you open your closet to choose your clothes for the day, do you see a collection of favorites hung on padded hangers or a crowded clump of "nothing to wear"?

- For breakfast, do you grab whatever's easy, or do you give some thought to making a nutritious blender drink or cooking oatmeal in an actual pot?

- Do you always take the same route to work, or do you spice it up sometimes and go through a part of town that's especially beautiful, or at least different?

Paying attention to questions like these can make art of your day before 9:00 A.M. Think of what you can do with sixteen waking hours! It is almost impossible to feel the empty yearning that leads to mindless eating or senseless spending when you're consciously involved in creating something. You are, you know, creating something all the time: your legacy.

Expect things to get far more interesting when you start treating every day, even Monday, as a venue for creative expression. Very little can be seen as ordinary when every choice, from the shoes you wear to the sandwich you order, is an opportunity to create a life that is, in one tiny way after another, ever more fascinating.

Take an Action

Be creative today—with the clothes you choose, the way you set the table, how you wrap a package. No aspect of life is too insignificant to count as art.

Chapter 6

YES, YOU'RE FLAWED.
AND YOU'RE PERFECT.
CHEW ON THAT

In order to feel full on the inside and live our visible lives as effectively as possible, every one of us has to come to grips with who we are. That's why we've heard from the Delphic oracle, "Man, know thyself," from Shakespeare, "This above all else, to thine own self be true," and from our best friend from eighth grade, "Get real."

Most people aren't clamoring to be first in the self-knowledge checkout line. We're afraid of what we might find out and prefer to remain giddily deluded. Throughout the ages, however, there have been men and women who, in the course of going about their business, bumped smack into self-knowledge (and into quite a few insights about life in general while they were at it). People who have received direct knowledge in this way we call *mystics*.

One definition of the word *mystic* is somebody who's on the woo-woo fringe—you know, the one who says, "For twenty bucks I'll tell your fortune, and for twenty thousand I'll cure your diseases." That's not a mystic; that's a con artist. Genuine mystics are individuals who have had an *experience* of the truth. They enter into a state of being in which all they have held as true steps aside long enough for them to come to another knowing, one more real than the book in your hand and your ability to read it.

Some of these people you've heard of: Jakob Boehme, the Baal Shem Tov, Catherine of Siena. Others have written poetry you've read for your own pleasure or because you had an English teacher who was in love with Wordsworth or Rumi, Whitman or Blake. Some used their experience to change society. Bill Wilson, for example, was a low-bottom drunk until he had a textbook-perfect mystical experience in the 1930s. After that, he never took another drink and went on to co-found Alcoholics Anonymous.

Most mystics, however, aren't known outside their time and their town. They're just people who stumble onto magnificence, and after they do, nothing is ever the same. They come from every religious tradition and from outside religious traditions. Gender, nationality, social status, and intelligence quotient (or devoutness quotient, for that matter) are of no consequence. What these people have in common is that they've been somewhere most of us will never go—the way you feel a strange camaraderie with someone who's been to Malawi or Bulgaria if you've been there too.

What the mystics say about the world is that it's right on schedule. Even the awful parts have a place in the plan, although we're still supposed to work with all that's in us to make things better. They implore us to get along, not just because it's a good idea but because they know that *there's only one of us here anyway*. Yep, we're all part of a piece. And if that isn't weird enough, they say that everything is made out of Love, or Light (synonyms these folks use a lot), and this Love or Light is what we're made out of too. We don't always seem like loving little sunbeams because we (our souls, to use a familiar term, as opposed to our ego-selves or personalities) opted to experience a plane of existence where having weaknesses shows us our strengths, and assorted overcomings bulk up our character. This is Planet Earth. Disneyland of the cosmos. The place to rock and roll, people.

First off, you get a body. The ancient Vedic texts of India claim that even the angels envy the human body because it can do so many things and through it we can experience such exquisite physical, emotional, and mental pleasures. There's a whole alphabet of them: amusement, arousal, à la mode; beauty, bliss, bonding; calmness, cheerfulness, cunnilingus—oops, I'll stop there, but you get what I'm saying.

There is a price, however, for these perks of life on earth: signing up to live here means coming into a world of opposites—night and day, hot and cold, happy and sad … you know, the bunch of them. In a world of opposites it's difficult to remain aware of the ultimate reality that there really is only one Power in the universe, the Beneficence that got us here in the first place. Thus (drumroll, please), the truth about you: you are flawed. As a human being, you come equipped with the same pairs of opposites as everything else on this planet. You're kind—and crabby. You're generous—and self-serving.

You made A's in math and history—and had to have a tutor for Spanish. Your flaws are part of the texture of your personality. You can work on them and improve some of them quite a bit. The rest you'll take to your grave. Other people (also flawed, by the way) will love you anyhow, and life is decidedly more pleasant if you can love yourself too.

Even though you are flawed in your human self, your personality-self, you are also perfect. I'm not talking about the perfect-hair, perfect-skin, perfect-abs, perfect-job, perfect-spouse, perfect-kids brand of perfection. This is about your *nature*, the reality of who you are that underlies and goes beyond your hair, skin, abs, job, spouse, kids, expectations, aspirations, and the rest. You are perfect because you are an expression of the Divine. You don't have to do anything or believe anything for this to be true. You don't even have to be aware of it, but if you are, you'll feel less emptiness and more power.

If the concept of being a perfect divine expression is new to you, or if it rubs uncomfortably against another belief you hold, just let it be for now. Eventually you'll figure out where to fit it amid all the concepts you've explored in your life, embracing some, discarding others.

In my case, the exploration started early. It surprised no one that I studied comparative religions in college since I'd grown up in a sort of United Nations of belief systems. My dad wanted me to be Catholic, so I went to Mass on Sundays and for "instruction" every Saturday morning. My mother wanted me to experience other churches (and synagogues and temples) so we went to all of them—at least all the ones they had in Kansas City at the time. Dede, the woman who lived with us to take care of me and who was, I see now, my first spiritual teacher, took me to her Unity church and regaled me with tales of Emerson, Mary Baker Eddy, and the Bhagavad Gita. The nuns weren't thrilled when I talked about reincarnation in catechism class, and I remember the reprimand I got for sharing what I thought was the edifying information that Krishna and Zarathushtra had virgin births too(!).

Although I can swap Sister-Mary-Josephine-was-mean stories with the best of them, she planted some exquisite ideas in my consciousness that have stayed with me to this day. One of them was her question, "From what did God create us?" Correct answer: "God created us from Himself." There was no other choice because God, by whatever name or conception, was all there was. Still is.

And that's how you—and all of us—got to be perfect. With all our flaws. We gave up being perfectly perfect and agreed to be only borderline-excellent in order to experience this life. This way we get to grow and learn and, in the soul sense, strive to get back to where we started as consciously perfect rather than unconsciously so.

The knowledge that you are flawed (because it's the only way human beings come) and yet perfect (because your essence can be nothing less) gives you permission to fully exhale. You can lean on the notion that you're part of something great and grand and good. Ideally, this knowledge will inspire you to go forward with the conviction that you have a place and a purpose that is uniquely yours. You don't have to have perfect hair-skin-abs-job-spouse-kids because you're already perfect in the only way you have to be and the only way you can be. Because this is the truth about you, you are fully entitled to the best *imperfect* hair-skin-abs-job-spouse-kids going, or something even better.

What to do with this flawed-but-perfect concept? Chew on it. Mull it over. Who you really are is an eternal idea, as perfect as the Mind that conceived it. Your body and brain and life experiences will never be as fabulous as that—this is earth, for heaven's sake—but the closer you get to realizing who you genuinely are, the closer to pretty darned amazing you'll be, in every aspect of your life every day you live.

Take an Action

Give some serious thought to what it could mean in your life to truly own that you can't make yourself perfect because you already are, *and* that you'll never be perfect in some *just-how-much-like-Nicole-Kidman-can-I-get?* judgment system. This should help you lighten up quite a bit.

Chapter 7

YOUR LIFE BELIEVES
EVERY WORD YOU SAY

Mom was on to something when she said, "If you can't say
something nice, don't say anything at all." Most of us
follow her advice when we're talking to other people. It's a
rare (and unpopular) individual who'll say to a friend or
stranger, "You are so stupid," "You're such a slob," or, "Those
pants make you look like the side of a house." Few of us, however, are above making such comments (or thinking them—
same thing) to ourselves, virtually guaranteeing a relationship
with fat, broke & lonely. This is a pity, especially since the
right words can help us break up for good.

You've heard those stories of tribal witch doctors who give
a person a "death stick" that is believed by all to bring about
the demise of its recipient. It is well documented that people
have indeed died from this kind of thought transfer. Even in
modern society, there is statistical likelihood that a person
given, say, six months to live will indeed pass away at almost

precisely the six-month mark. Words, and the beliefs they engender, do have power. We can use this to our benefit or detriment.

Pay attention to what you're saying and notice when it diminishes your worth or your prospects. If you doubt the power of words, think back to your own childhood and bring to mind the one negative comment made to you by a parent or other authority figure that still trips you up today. Everybody I've polled on this subject has one: "You'll never be as pretty as your sister.... Girls aren't supposed to be good at math.... You're just not college material.... You can never expect a man to stay around.... Of course you're going to law school...."

When we're young and impressionable, we can grab on to a sentence like one of these and turn it into a life sentence, our inalterable destiny. Words affect us when we're older too, especially the ones that come out of our own mouths. Every time you give an unwanted situation credence by repeating it ("I hate it that I've gained all this weight.... I'll never get a job that pays enough.... Nobody will ever love me again"), it's as if you highlight that single aspect of your multifaceted being with an iridescent marker. On the page of your life, it's the only line that shows. It gives what was a manageable and changeable fact the status of immutable truth.

You change this pattern by changing your words. Be aware of what you say and get in the habit of doing a reframe/refocus every time you say something you wish you hadn't. Listen especially to your habitual phrases: "He's a pain in the butt.... I thought I was going to have a heart attack.... If it's not one thing it's another.... I knew it was too good to be true." It is *not* too good to be true. You decide the limits of good in your life, and if you're like most people, you've limited it way too much. Instead, let your words open the way to more of what you want and less of what you don't.

When someone says, "How are you?" try saying, "Terrific ... never better ... absolutely fabulous, and isn't this a beautiful day?" Now, you may be on the verge of barfing, and you suspect that I'm Pollyanna writing under a pseudonym, but look around you: positive people have better lives. If being positive does not come naturally to you, I empathize: it doesn't come naturally to me either, but neither do most of the other good habits that have helped me dump fat, broke & lonely. Besides, you can change your nature. Doing something long enough—whether it's getting up early or giving a cheery response to "How are you?"—makes inroads in your psyche until what once seemed strained becomes simply the way of things.

As you bring more affirmative words into your life, don't get caught in the trap of believing that in speaking positively you're not being honest. You could argue that position if words only reported circumstances, but they do more than that: they create circumstances. Therefore, "Everything is great" is just as true as "I'm getting a headache, I'm way behind on a report for my boss, and the guy who cut my hair this time should never have been allowed to graduate from beauty school."

Some people, especially women, are also wary of speaking positively because they feel that doing so is making too much of themselves. Despite our valiant history marked by suffragettes and bra-burners, the "good girl" messages persist. Decide today to take your place as a wonderful woman instead of a good girl. Claim your power, claim your success, and claim your place in this world by speaking up for yourself, owning the terrific things you've already brought into being, and allowing for those yet to come.

One caveat (the pearls-before-swine thing): when you are around men and women who adore negativity, who love awful-izing and rehashing the failings and misfortunes of family members, coworkers, and celebrities, say as little as possible. These are the people who are likely to respond to a possibility-laden statement such as "I'm planning to start my own business" with, "Well, you know, most new businesses fail." In the company of such down-in-the-mouthers, refuse to join the doomsaying and don't give them the chance to infect your best intentions with their negativity virus. There are times when silence makes an eloquent statement.

Take an Action

Start speaking positively, even if it makes you feel as if you're lying or speaking a foreign language in which you're nowhere near fluent. When you hear yourself say something negative, stop and rephrase it, whether it was verbalized or simply thought. Pay particular attention to recurring phrases, as in "My job makes me sick," or, "I'm at the end of my rope."

Chapter 8

GOT GOD*?

I'm giving God* an asterisk because so many people have trouble with the word. If you're one of them, think synonyms. A few of the myriad names God* answers to are:

- Life

- Light

- Love

- Higher Power

- The Divine

- Creator

- Source

- Goddess

- Spirit

- Universal Energy

- Presence

- Tao

- The Infinite

- The Force (from *Star Wars*), or the acronym some people swear by:

- **G**ood **O**rderly **D**irection

If these, like the G-word itself, seem to you to come with more baggage than your last boyfriend, remember that God-with-baggage has to do with ideologies and religions and the need that a lot of folks have to impose their views on everybody else. Filling your emptiness has nothing to do with ideology, and it has to do with religion only in the broadest sense of the term: its Latin root, *religare*, "to lead back." You want to be led back to knowing that God (Allah, Tao, whatever-you-want-to-call-it) is inside you. It is your essence. It is the spark that animates you and inspires your best intentions. It's always there. When you know that, you feel safe and sufficient.

People usually talk about God in the context of belief. For ending the tyranny of fat, broke & and lonely, though, what you believe is your business. It's what you know that counts, and what you can come to know is that this Force is with you every nanosecond of your life.

Still, the word *God* can be a hang-up. I once gave a full-day training on holistic health and self-care to the municipal employees of a prosperous suburb of Kansas City. The day before the event, the meeting planner e-mailed me something that, at first glance, looked like a vocabulary test from fifth grade. It was a two-column list of words I was not to say (column one) and those that were acceptable (column two). I could, for instance, say "fresh," but not "organic," and I could say "vegetable," but not "vegetarian." When it came to God, I couldn't say anything. Uttering "God," she explained, could offend the nonreligious, but something like "Universe" or "Higher Power" could offend the religious. I did the training day, albeit under a theistic (and agricultural) gag order.

Maybe you agree with her. You could be thinking, "I don't believe in God. This looked like a secular book and you flippin' tricked me." Or you could be coming from a completely different place: "Don't tell me about God. I know about God. And I can already tell you're some kind of weird hippie heathen, so there."

Look, we all have ideas about the Big Picture. Some of us believe there isn't one. You go around once. You do the best you can. Your kids and their kids and whatever good you've been able to do in this world will be left when you go, and that's enough. Besides, eighty years on earth is the best ride in the park.

Others of us espouse our understanding of a particular religion, the one our parents gave us or one we found ourselves. We might say, "I'm a born-again Christian," or, as I once saw on a T-shirt, "I'm a Buddhist—born again and again and again...." But even within religions there are countless ways of seeing what the founder of that religion taught.

One of my pet peeves, for example, is that the word *Chris-*
tian, which by definition should apply to anyone attempting
to follow the teachings of Jesus, is rapidly becoming the sole
province of only one brand of Christianity, evangelical, leav-
ing millions of Christ's flock semantically stranded. I was
shocked to hear one of my daughter's friends say, "Catholics
aren't supposed to use birth control, but it's okay for Chris-
tians." I couldn't help tossing in my sarcastic two cents: "Gosh,
somebody had better tell the pope he's not a Christian. I'll bet
anything he didn't know."

Some people find meaning in life by constructing a
worldview of their own out of bits and pieces from phi-
losophies and religions and personal revelations. Others
infuse their base path with an auxiliary one—there are so
many Jewish people practicing Buddhism, for instance, that
someone even came up with the term "Jew-Bu" to describe
them. This mixing and matching that once would have
been unheard of, even considered blasphemous, isn't just
possible now—it's necessary. If the teachings of Judaism,
Christianity, and Sufism, the mystical arm of Islam, can exist
in harmony in the life of even one individual, that's a micro-
cosmic picture of those three faiths existing in harmony on
one planet.

Obviously, you don't have to feel overly responsible for
peace in the Middle East just because you don't want to be
fat, broke & lonely. It's just that, because everything is connected, coming to know that the Divine owns real estate in
your heart and soul brings your life to a higher level. That el-
evates all life, even if just a little. And when you know without question that the Divine is inside you, you can't help but

realize that it's in everybody else too—even when it doesn't seem to show much.

Here's the deal: if living on your own power isn't getting you where you want to be, get connected to a Power that can go the distance for you—a Power that's greater than your ego and yet resides within you as the very substance of your being. You don't have to sign anything or join anything. You might simply say something like, "Okay, my life is kind of screwed up, and I don't even know who I'm talking to, but if there's more inside me than I've been aware of and it can fill me up today, I'll take it. And thanks."

That ought to do it. Make special note of the word *today*. It's important. God (and now that we understand each other, let's retire the asterisk) operates in the present tense. It's "Give us this day our daily bread," not "Please make sure I have two loaves of pumpernickel a week from Thursday." Making contact daily—and sometimes more than that—is essential. You might ask in the morning to feel secure and satisfied and to know that you're enough, yet by noon feel the emptiness eating at you just the same. If that happens, check in again. If this is new to you, it will take some time. Just keep coming back to the idea that you can feel safe. And filled up. And that even when you don't feel like it, you really are enough.

Take an Action

If you guys aren't well acquainted, get tight with God—in a way that feels comfortable and lets you be yourself. If you have a less than idyllic relationship, get right with God. Maybe you'll need to devise a more loving, friendly, and accessible image than the one somebody gave you a long time ago. If the whole God thing is a deal-breaker for you, come up with another concept of a power beyond your ego that you can plug into and draw strength from. This might be nature, the flow of life, the bond of love—whatever works.

Chapter 9

WHEN DOING NOTHING CAN GIVE YOU EVERYTHING

A while back, I took an inventory of my professional life. On the left-hand side of the page I wrote every noteworthy success I'd experienced up until then. On the right-hand side I wrote what I'd done to bring about each red-letter event. The right-hand column was most illuminating: every entry said either "nothing" or "I showed up."

It wasn't that I'd been sitting around watching TV and waiting for miracles. I did my daily tasks. When I wrote a book or article or when I gave a talk, I gave it everything I had, but every major "break" came from out of the ever-so-accommodating blue. No manipulating, strategizing, or finagling required. In fact, my best-laid plans and manipulations have, for the most part, fallen on their manipulative faces. I've pretty much given up on them.

What this shows me is that we can't force anything. Instead, our job is to keep the path cleared for the good stuff to ride in on. Like an isometric exercise, this may look like doing nothing. *Nothing*, however, involves holding the vision of what we want, staying confident (even when that's a stretch), doing what's required in the moment, and tuning in to that barely perceptible inner voice and acting on what it says. This last piece is doing nothing *cum laude*.

The crowning glory of productive inactivity, meditation or contemplation, can dispatch inner emptiness more effectively than any other single method. If you charge your cell phone, program your coffee maker, and gas up your tank, you already know that a full battery, Colombian dark roast, and unleaded regular are essential to the way you live. Concentrated nothing-doing—sitting in a chair or on the floor in total silence appearing to be, oh my gosh, *wasting time*—does for you as a human entity what you do so automatically for the various machines in your life: it powers you up.

So here's what you do: nothing! Well, almost. You get up in the morning and light a little candle on the table by your bed as a reminder that you're not going to jump into your day without charging your soul. To do this you sit—on the bed leaning against the headboard, on the floor cross-legged with your back against the bed or the wall, or in a chair with both feet on the floor and your hands resting comfortably in your lap. Close your eyes and notice the remarkable fact that you just keep breathing—which is evidence in itself that you have a reason to be here; otherwise, why wouldn't your breathing just stop?

Once you've tuned in to the rhythm of your breathing, match a silent affirmation to it. Inhale "I am ..." and exhale "... enough." Or inhale "God ..." and exhale "... loves me."

Or (this is the one I use) inhale "All is ..." and exhale "... well." You can use any short phrase you like as long as it's positive and something with which you sincerely wish to program your mind. Sit there and do this for ten or fifteen or twenty minutes. Twenty is a little better than ten and ten is enormously better than blowing this off.

You'll have all sorts of extraneous thoughts ("Is the sprinkler on?" "Do I have clean socks?" "This is dull—why am I doing it?"). Don't fight the thoughts, but don't entertain them either. Just give each one a nod and let it float by like a wispy white cloud in an otherwise clear sky. Then come back to your phrase and your breath.

Do this every morning. If you miss a morning, don't miss the next one. For even more benefit, meditate again in the early evening—either by staying late at work, if there's a private corner in your office, or by doing another ten, fifteen, or twenty minutes of meditation when you get home. This can be a lovely way to punctuate the divide between your workday and your private life. Bottom line: meditating twice a day is terrific, but meditating once a day is indispensable.

Here's what's in it for you:

- *Fullness:* After you've done this for a while and get the hang of it, you'll feel less needy about whatever it is you've been needing.

- *Calmness:* Someone like me (Aries and half Italian) is never going to be nonstop placid, but the degree of calmness in anyone's life increases with regular meditation.

- *Insights:* Since you're opening the channels to the best that's inside you (you'll sometimes see this called your *higher self*), little brilliances will just pop up in a way they didn't before. They'll come in the form of solutions to problems or as creative ideas. Some of these will just give you a better day. One or two of them might give all of us a better world.

Regular meditation also purportedly has a plethora of health benefits: lower blood pressure, reduced cholesterol, fewer sick days, a slowing of the aging process. You get the perks, of course, only if you do the practice. That takes commitment and discipline. If you've been short on those, this is a nice, gentle place to learn them. Of course, if you'd rather learn the hard way, that option is always available. I suggest that you make it easy on yourself and begin the ageless art of focused non-doing this afternoon or first thing tomorrow. Keep it up, and fat, broke & lonely won't have a chance.

Take an Action

Sit in silence for at least ten minutes within the next twenty-four hours. Intend to repeat this practice daily until you're older than you ever thought you'd get. If at first you're bored or this practice doesn't seem to be doing anything, that's fine. You're doing it exactly right.

Chapter 10

FIT, FLUSH, PARTNERED & STILL EMPTY IS JUST FAT, BROKE & LONELY IN DRAG

Deepening your inner life is imperative for making the break from fat, broke & lonely. You didn't go to all the trouble to get yourself a life on earth, put your mother through labor, and endure toilet training, the multiplication tables, and middle school in order to spend your adult life dealing with fat, broke & lonely, or even one member of the group.

You were created to be happy, healthy, and pleased with yourself. You're supposed to have all you need and the motivation to work for more—for yourself and your family first, then for those who can use some help. You're supposed to be liked, loved, and respected and to have people in your life whom you like, love, and respect. When you know this, and live each day remembering that you know it, you're free.

And that's the crux of it: freedom. Liberation. Not losing weight (again) or paying off your debt so you can charge some more. Freedom. You know, like "We pledge ... our Lives, our Fortunes, and our sacred Honor," and, "Free at last! Thank God Almighty, we are free at last!" I am not using these allusions lightly or with any disrespect: I really mean that attaining this degree of freedom is what breaking up with fat, broke & lonely is all about.

Years ago, in a support group for people with food issues, I had a mentor, Ellen, who was quite a bit older than me. She had kept her weight off for a long time and was invariably able to speak to my condition with some maxim of her own creation: "Fear is fattening," or, "When you change one part of your life, it will touch every part."

We lived on different sides of town and I didn't see Ellen often, but we talked a few times a week, except when her husband answered and said that she was in too much pain from her arthritis to come to the phone. After not seeing Ellen for about six months, I ran into her at a conference and saw that she had gained some thirty pounds. I was shocked and felt betrayed. How could this woman, with all her wise words, be having a clandestine affair with Baskin-Robbins and not tell me?

After a little uncomfortable small talk, I made my excuses and went off to look for someone who also knew Ellen, so I could express my dismay and gossip with complete justification. I chose a woman named Donna to be my comrade in character assassination. She declined. "Vicki [see, I told you this was years ago], Ellen is on heavy steroids for her arthritis. That's where the weight came from. She only looks fat. She's really free."

Just as Ellen's appearance of bondage was deceiving, it is also possible—and common—to give the appearance of freedom but still be enslaved. You can be thin because you're bulimic. Or addicted to dieting and too much exercise. Or even suffering from some terrible disease that you'd give anything to be rid of, regardless of how much you'd weigh without it. You can have money because you stole it. Or because you stockpile it like a modern-day Ebenezer Scrooge. You could be the most popular girl in town, but surrounded by fair-weather friends who'd disappear if you fell on hard times. You might be in a relationship that looks just ducky—because no one knows your guy is jealous, controlling, or even abusive.

In other words, you can be fit, flush, and partnered and still empty on the inside. Afraid. Dejected. Spinning your wheels to keep up appearances because that way you're at least keeping up. Maybe you've been there. Maybe you are there. If so, you have plenty of company. Too many people are holding things together for appearance's sake but lack the foundation of an intact spirit.

We're invariably taken aback when someone with a "perfect" life breaks down, becomes depressed, or has a midlife crisis, whether they're middle-aged or some other age. This is because we believe what we see. When we look at somebody who is fat, broke & lonely, we know they'd like things to be different, but when the fit, flush, and partnered fall apart, it seems to defy logic. Keep in mind, however, that inner emptiness can show—or not. It may, in fact, be at its most insidious when it is well camouflaged by good looks, success, a lovely family, and enviable social status. It shouldn't be there. But it is.

What looks like an exemplary life on the outside may be the result of filling the empty spaces through self-knowledge and living in integrity. Or this appearance could come from simply covering up the empty spaces and, in the denial, deepening them. In other words, we may be looking at an attractive life that's for real, one built on a firm foundation, or not for real, one built on sand and sham. All the pieces are there, but there's nothing shoring them up. The tiniest gust could bring the whole thing down.

Therein lies the danger, as the saying goes, of comparing your insides to someone else's outsides. Emptiness, whether overt or concealed, begs to be filled. The appearance of fit, flush, and partnered is good as far as it goes, but it can be a ruse—fat, broke & lonely in drag. Anyone can gain weight, lose money, end a relationship, fall out of favor. Often this is because they can no longer pedal fast enough to maintain the charade. Sometimes, as in Ellen's case, the appearance changes because life takes detours beyond human control.

Either way, you'll go further if you refuse to waste energy envying someone who seems to have it all together or feeling smugly superior to someone who seems not to. It's fine to learn from people you admire, but don't put them on pedestals. Pedestals are for busts, not whole human beings who are complex mixtures of heaven and earth, altruism and egotism, unassailable intentions and, sometimes, unfortunate choices. Keep your focus on your own life and on the task at hand: getting yourself together from your innermost soul on out. The desire for externals like an athletic body or the enticing trinkets that money can buy does have motivational value. That's fine, as long as you don't confuse the externals with the eternals.

Before going forward in this book with the specific strategies for dealing with fat, broke, and lonely as individual issues and taking the necessary steps to give your life more depth and breadth and purpose, be sure that you've made a reasonable start on developing, or strengthening, your inner life. Look back over the action steps in this section. If you haven't taken them, do. And consciously incorporate the ongoing actions into your way of thinking and your way of being. Are you coming to grips with essential emptiness? Are you paying attention to the words you choose? Have you started meditating? These actions may not seem aggressive enough to face fat, broke & lonely, but they are your front line. Without them, either you'll make no progress at all or you'll make it to fit, flush, and partnered and lose them to the cavernous and consuming gap inside you.

Although "having it all" may sound like leftover greed from the dot-com era, you should, in this context, expect to have it all. You're going for not just fit, flush, partnered, and popular, but for a meaningful life that supports and sustains a healthy body, a healthy bottom line, and healthy relationships. Don't skimp on the foundation. This is not about a smaller-size dress from a more expensive store. It's about developing a way of living that, as the natural way of things, leads to your fitting into the size you want, shopping at the store you want, and wearing what you bought there in the company of the people you want to be around. When you have the basics down, this happy scenario isn't some temporary aberration ("Let's have fun now—this can't last") but simply the way your life works. Fit, flush, and partnered? More than likely. Scared you'll screw up and lose them all? Not even a little.

Take an Action

Observe people you know and people you read about or see on TV who seem to have it all together. Who do you think looks good but is really fit, flush, partnered, and still empty? How can you tell? Choose your role models carefully. You don't want to hitch your wagon to any falling stars.

Part Two

BREAKING UP WITH FAT

There is a power inside you that leads to right decisions, even in areas as ordinary as your food choices and getting to the gym.

Having a food or weight problem is an opportunity to get in touch with the wisdom and power inside you. You'll need that wisdom and power to make the right choices at breakfast, lunch, and dinner and to stay on track when you pass a bakery or see an ad for some superburger.

Food is supposed to be delicious (whether you're thin, fat, or think you're fat). Your body is supposed to be luscious, whether you are naturally angular, muscular, or curvy. Movement is supposed to be *play*, the way it is for kids and puppies. Your ego-self may not always see things this way, but your higher self does. Your part is to go along with that, to enjoy eating and moving and living in a body.

Some of the chapters that follow deal with off-the-shelf fat—the kind that comes from rich food and a desk job—and others focus on the inner emptiness that some of us have tried (quite understandably, if you think about it) to fill with food. Read them all. Apply in your life those that apply to your life.

Chapter 11

FAT *PHOBIA* MAY ALSO BE HARMFUL TO YOUR HEALTH

Everybody knows that being too fat is bad for your health. But so is being scared to death of it. Our society is schizophrenic about the whole issue. On the one hand, we've collaborated with our cars, TVs, and computers, our fast food, processed food, and ever-available food, to become a nation in which the majority of us are overweight. But as a nation in which the majority is supposed to rule, we've also demonized fat and the people wearing it. We regard fat as shameful, even disgusting. What a setup for the kind of self-hatred that a good old chocolate shake could take care of!

If you want the skinny on fat, this is it: it's as much a cultural construct as an anatomical reality. The fat on your body is stored energy, stored fuel. In an evolutionary sense, those of us with the ability to store fat efficiently were the lucky ones: we survived the famines to eulogize all those model-and-ballerina types who just couldn't last them out.

But every bit as real as the love handle you can get your hands on is how differently that love handle is viewed in different eras and societies. Several years ago I saw on an international satellite station a Tahitian news anchor, male, who weighed at least four hundred pounds—substantially over the max to qualify for an anchor job here. "Fattening camps" still exist in Mauritania, and young girls are sent there to be force-fed rich foods so they'll be plump enough to compete in the marriage market. The Renaissance ideal was today's Lane Bryant shopper. The "bathing beauties" of the early twentieth century were short and curvy ("oh, what five-foot-two can do …"), while the fashion ideal of the sixties was skinny and flat-chested. It's still pretty thin, but through the miracle of plastic surgery, it's now skinny with boobs.

The issue, then, isn't just how much fat is on your body, but when and where your body happens to show up. I know you want to lose your extra weight, and I applaud that, but a vital step toward that goal is to get clear on the fact that somewhere your body type—even if you detest it—is considered beautiful and desirable. There is a woman somewhere who would give anything for your body (or the one you're scared to death you might grow into). A plus-sized friend of mine was practically stalked in rural India by women wanting to know her secret for being "so fat and so beautiful." They lamented that as hard as they tried, they just couldn't accomplish what she had.

To be free of fat (or an obsession with it), you have to desensitize yourself on the subject and get to a place of emotional neutrality. This does not mean giving up or giving in, but rather detaching from the strong opinions many of us have about weight. To reach this neutral state, make a study of fat the way a scientist would study some phenomenon to which he has absolutely no personal attachment. Do this by looking at paintings, looking at people, and looking into the way fat is regarded in cultures around the world. Fat or thin needs to become like turquoise or aqua, Pepsi or Coke—you might prefer one over the other, but the difference is slight.

The aim of this desensitization is to shed your anxiety about gaining weight, or not losing the weight you have gained, or some variation on the theme. Fear is like rubber cement: it keeps you stuck to what you're afraid of. Besides, fat has a curious penchant for returning to those who are afraid of it.

Once the steamer trunk full of judgments that you hold about fat (ugly, lazy, dirty, sexless, slutty, grotesque, and all the rest) gets tossed overboard, you can look dispassionately at your own body and at the phenomenon of overweight and obesity in the affluent world. If you want to lose some fat and replace it with hard-earned muscle, you'll be losing *fat*, not ugliness, laziness, dirt, sexlessness, sluttiness, or grotesqueness—because you didn't have those to begin with.

Then you can go beyond your body to see who you really are: you are not your body. You are the essence that animates it, that twenty-one grams you'll lose someday when you leave here and go on to the next adventure. J. Krishnamurti described it beautifully in his little classic of the spiritual life, *At the Feet of the Master*. He wrote: "Your body is your animal, the horse upon which you ride. Therefore, you must treat it well, not overwork it, you must feed it properly on pure food and drink only.... But it must always be you who controls that body, not it that controls you."

For me, this makes the whole weight issue less personal and subsequently less daunting. I am perfect and so are you (remember chapter 6 about being flawed and perfect at the same time?). The agents of fat, broke & lonely—people and companies that stand to gain either from the consumption required to keep you fat or the expenditures inherent in the repeated quest for getting thin—are betting that you'll never depart from the belief that you're a mess. Otherwise the junk food wouldn't look so good, the diet stuff wouldn't be such a draw, and you wouldn't be such a ready consumer of processed foods; weight-loss programs, pills, and provisions; a wardrobe that spans five sizes; and the deserted exercise equipment that looked so cool on the infomercial. (If you really want the exercise gear, get it on eBay or at a yard sale. There's tons of it out there, and you'll save a mint.)

Way back in chapter 2, I gave you a basic metaphysical principle: what you focus on is what comes into your life. Now you can apply that principle in a practical way. You have to stop focusing on fat, hating it, fearing it, and fighting it. Instead, you're going to be focusing on your own worth and beauty and on the Power inside you that can do what your exhausted willpower can't. The first step, however, isn't to change your body. It's to appreciate it.

Take an Action

Move beyond your fear of fat. Look at the Old Masters' paintings of voluptuous bodies and at photographs of the woman-shaped screen goddesses from the forties and fifties. Admire the work of singers and actresses who aren't thin without uttering the caveat: "If she'd only lose some weight...." Admire yourself, your body, and your being today, without the caveat "If I'd only lose some weight...."

Chapter 12

START SEEING YOURSELF AS GORGEOUS. NOW

I was a kid when Muhammad Ali, then Cassius Clay, started spouting, "I am the greatest." It was revolutionary at the time. Nobody said things like that, and it made some folks uncomfortable. I heard grown-ups mumble, "He can't really mean that." Well, he did. And he went on to prove it. I invite you to do the same thing.

Start seeing yourself as magnificent, and your body as gorgeous, right now, this minute, whether you want to keep it as is or help it to a higher degree of strength and health by making certain changes in its care and feeding. In the meantime, if anybody tells you that you are not gorgeous, they're just plain wrong. What I really want to say is, whoever doesn't think you're splendid precisely as you are is not a person you need in your life. If it's a guy, leave the jerk!—in a few years he'll have a paunch of his own to worry about. If it's the father of your children and you're not going anywhere, at least don't internalize the criticisms—and this holds true whether they come from a husband, lover, sister, mom, or anybody else.

Maybe you're thinking, "But I really am fat. It's not healthy. I could die. Anyone who really loves me will tell me that." No. You just told yourself that, and you probably do it several times a day. You already know how much you weigh, your pants size, your measurements, and probably some skin-pinched approximation of your BMI (body mass index, the percentage of fat in your body). These numbers may be hard to take, but they're only numbers—and in almost every case they're changeable, with your cooperation. Your cooperation will not be forthcoming because people around you berate you. It will come when your own self-estimation rises to that of someone who's willing to make changes. The first change required of you? To see yourself as gorgeous.

To come to the belief that you are indeed gorgeous *right now*, you can do mental exercises such as reciting affirmations ("I am exquisite just the way I am"), putting little signs around as reminders ("You're totally worth it: don't forget"), or playing self-hypnosis audios that will tell you this stuff for forty minutes. Whether you're the self-hypnosis type or not, you must take the very pragmatic step of treating yourself as someone extraordinary. It doesn't matter if you don't believe it yet; you just have to act as if you do. Don't tell me you can't do that: you've sucked up to bosses you didn't really respect and batted your eyelashes at guys you weren't all that interested in. This "acting as if" is simply re-routing a little respect and admiration in your own direction.

Some ways to start include:

- Buy something new to wear—before you lose an ounce.

- Get some nice exercise attire: you don't even have to exercise right now, just have the clothes for it.

- Get a professional makeup job (a cosmetic-counter makeover counts).

- Have a manicure and pedicure—paid for at a salon, bartered with a friend, or self-service.

- Clear the ratty stuff out of your lingerie drawer and replace at least some of the discards with nice, new pieces.

Lingerie is a big deal—bras, panties, camisoles, the stuff you sleep in, all of it. You think nobody sees it (although in recent years we've been seeing it quite a bit), but even if you're single and celibate and you've never revealed a thong or a bra strap to the innocent public, there is one person who sees your underwear: you.

They said in the Great Depression, "It's honorable to wear patches." That may be, but reserve them for jackets and jeans and keep your unmentionables above reproach. The state of your nightwear will affect the attitude you have when you awaken. The condition of the clothing closest to your skin will subtly influence the way you treat yourself all day (including your eating and exercise choices). Designer duds are not necessary. Your undies just have to be nice. How nice?

Nice enough that if your regular guy morphed into a heart-throb of the silver screen, you'd feel good in your underwear.

Although the lingerie drawer is of primary importance, get around to cleaning out other drawers and cupboards and cabinets and files—not all at once (that's purge mentality), but a little at a time. *You are gorgeous* and in every way deserving of good things. Everything you look at and interact with on a regular basis—your wardrobe, your house or apartment, your desk at work, your car—needs to be in a state that's attractive and functional. When your environment is suitable for someone of value and worth, it helps you see yourself as that person.

Celebrate yourself. Don't wait for some guy to send you flowers. Get yourself flowers. (That might even alert the guy that you actually *like* flowers. Who'd have thought?) Use the good dishes even when you're just having lunch by yourself. You'll feel better. (The plate alone can affect what you put on it: it's just weird to stick cold pizza or a couple of Twinkies on your grandmother's china.) Reframe mundane chores into opportunities for self-care: you're making the bed because you deserve to have a lovely place to come home to; you're washing the windows to let the sun shine in and because it's good feng shui.

You see, dear reader (I never thought I'd say "dear reader," but it just felt right), you came forth because Life craved expression, and It made the divine decision to express as you. You! So, you may want to lose some weight. Fine. You may well be happier after that and healthier too, but *losing weight will not alter your worth.*

We all know that beauty is in the eye of the beholder. If

beauty is not what you behold when you look at yourself, you can do things to alter the image—eat differently, exercise, invest in flattering clothes, even get some surgical tweak if you're of a mind to. But start right now changing the eye that beholds the image. Without this internal, attitudinal eyelift, other transformations aren't going to make much difference.

Take an Action

Decide that you are absolutely gorgeous as you are and support your decision with acts of self-care. If you'd prefer to exist on five hundred calories and perform five hundred crunches, that's your clue that self-punishment is familiar and self-appreciation isn't. Nevertheless, in the next seventy-two hours, do at least two of the following: buy yourself something new to wear; clear out your lingerie drawer; straighten another drawer, cupboard, or file; get a massage or a salon service; give yourself flowers; or do something just for fun—a boat ride, a beach walk, a chick flick, whatever would make you happy.

Chapter 13

WHAT YOU'RE LOOKING FOR IS NOT IN THE REFRIGERATOR

I researched this chapter for thirty-two years. That's how long I spent either eating for a fix or dieting with a vengeance, carrying extra weight or knowing I would again as soon as the diet du jour wore off, which it always did. Happily, I can report that it's been over twenty years since my last binge. This gives me sufficient credentials to make this statement: if you're someone who uses food the way I did, what you're looking for is not in the refrigerator. It only seems that way because extra food can make you feel better for a little while. So can crack, I understand. It's in the long run that they turn on you.

In an archival family album, a black-and-white photograph shows me at my first birthday party, lunging for the cake. I wasn't reaching or stretching or flailing in babyish bliss toward something new and interesting. I knew it was cake. I was quite precocious when it came to desserts. Anyway, I was lunging at cake before I could walk steadily, and in between diets I continued lunging at any sweet, salty, or simply solid comestible for the next three decades.

Making the tale more tantalizing to share with the various experts I went to for help was the fact that my father was a doctor who had steered his practice away from ear, nose, and throat and toward shots, pills, and diets. I needed no teenage forays into illegal drugs; I'd been on intermittently prescribed speed since I was ten. My mom was in the anti-fat business for a time too. She worked in "reducing salons"—pre–health club establishments that featured machines with belts and rollers that look comical now but in their day seemed deadly serious. When I was about five, she and my dad opened a re-ducing salon of their own. They never said, "Hide! You're bad for business," but parents don't have to say everything aloud for a kid to get the message.

The diets my folks put me on then, and the ones I put myself on later, gave any rich, gooey, heavy food an allure far beyond what it could merit on its own. It was the great white hope (or, sometimes, the great chocolate hope) promising to give me peace when I was agitated, comfort when I was scared, and, years later, the means to get through a boring af-ternoon at my boring job or a long night in my lonely apart-ment. But all it gave me was something to focus on while I was eating it. The lump it put in my stomach didn't eradicate the knot of discomfort that was already there. It just moved over. Then I had a rock and a hard place—my own personal cliché just below the waistband of my jeans.

So here's what happened: I got so tired of fighting that the battle fatigue became worse than the cravings. I was, quite literally, fed up. At age thirty-three, for one amazing instant, I didn't care if I was fat or thin. I just had to get out from under. I said that to God, and probably because I really meant it, God seemed to say, "Okay. I've been waiting for you to come around." I decided to give the Power that had sustained me all along the opportunity to get me from lunch to dinner without a Snickers bar.

I found people who'd broken free before me, and I got their help. I didn't binge and I didn't diet—but only from morning to night, because that was as long I could do it. I joined a gym but refused to state a "goal weight," because I saw for the first time that my goal had to be health and sanity and a purposeful life. Anything else could come up and hit me from behind. With a giant cinnamon roll.

I'm at a different stage of life now, but what worked then still does. Menopause, the supreme stand-off between Woman, who's just getting her bearings, and Nature, who's done with her, changed the shape of my body some, but my weight stays pretty steady. I don't have cravings like I used to. Every now and then I eat too much at a meal. That doesn't ruin everything or blow anything. These days, eating too much, like arriving late for an appointment or turning in an article with an uncorrected typo, is evidence of my human-ness. Perfection is not a prerequisite for being able to stay at the weight I like, eat the food I like, and not obsess over either one.

Maybe you don't relate to the kind of compulsive eating I turned into a twisted art form. Still, if you ever eat in a way that gives you remorse (or indigestion), if you lust after food (or fearfully avoid it), if you look at fruit or a salad and think,

"Yeah, but where's the real food?" you would do well to internalize the fact that what you are looking for is not in the refrigerator. Or on the menu. Or at the market. Even though
men and women employ myriad filler behaviors to deal with
the empty hole inside, eating is the most obvious. You feel
empty. You try to fill it with something that's pleasant going
down and substantial once it gets there. But unlike physical
hunger, this emptiness is in your soul, and that's not part of
the digestive system.

What you're looking for is not in the refrigerator. It's in you,
deep inside, in your connection to a Higher Power and a higher
purpose. Once you get that, you start to fill your life with color
and delight, passion and commitment. Everything becomes
more delicious, food included, because you slow down and
savor it as one of the perks of life on earth, but only one of so
many you couldn't exhaust them if you lived to be 110.

Do this:

- *Drill yourself on "What you're looking for is not in the
  refrigerator"* as if that were the one fact that would ace a
  critical exam.

- *Get together with your Higher Power.* Say something like,
  "You know, this eating deal has pretty much got me.
  Would you just take it today and let me live my life?
  Thanks. I appreciate it."

- *Put yourself first.* This may seem at odds with being
  "spiritual," but damn it, you're a person too. Don't let
  responding to the needs of everybody else get in the
  way of meeting your own needs.

- *Keep company with people who can actually help.* I recommend Overeaters Anonymous (www.overeatersanonymous. org). It costs nothing and everybody's welcome, whether you're overweight, underweight, or whatever. There are no scales there and no diets, and they've got the twelve-step program that deals with addictions the way garlic and a crucifix take care of vampires.

- *Get rid of your scale.* You have been focused on your body for far too long. Focus on your life, of which your body is a reflection. Make changes there. The physical changes will follow—maybe not for your high school reunion or this year's swimsuit season, but for keeps.

This is probably a different way of dealing with the fat issue than you're used to. Good. Those other ways haven't worked. It's time to be radical. And willing. And brave. And ready to fly. I mean, isn't that what you came here for?

Take an Action

If you have an eating problem, follow up on every bullet point in this chapter, including locating Overeaters Anonymous in your area. You may think you have all sorts of convincing reasons for why you shouldn't do that, but you really have only one: you don't want to stop eating for a fix. Face that and go to a meeting anyway. Do what the people there tell you. Get this monkey off your back so you can help somebody else do it too. If you don't have an eating problem, develop compassion for those who do.

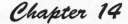

Chapter 14

FILL YOUR LIFE,
THEN YOUR PLATE

Overeating is a direct corollary to underliving. Oh, I know there are lots of reasons why people get fat: fast food, junk food, snacking, sodas, sitting all day, driving everywhere, spending evenings with the high-definition hypnotist, and getting locked into a diet/pork-out cycle that confuses the body and makes losing weight more difficult. Despite these disparate causes, however, a sizable portion of the solution lies in living fully, with your priorities straight, your talents in use, and your passions engaged. When your life is filled with meaning and purpose and fun and games (especially the kind that make you sweat), you may not be skinny—who needs skinny anyway?—but you should no longer have to worry about being fat.

You'd think that for anyone not dealing with war, poverty, or a debilitating disease, living a big, juicy life would be the norm. Instead, such lives are exceptional. They're noted in the media, which has been known to stretch and spin certain lives to look bigger and juicier than they actually are because we want so much to read and hear about them. The convenient mythology is that having a big, juicy life calls for being a superhuman human with more beauty, brains, and lean muscle mass than a mere mortal dares to hope for. Baloney. There's a big, juicy life out there with your name on it. Claim it by saying yes to opportunities, committing to getting more out of life in April than you did in March, and living in color instead of black and white (photographic exhibitions and classic films exempted, of course).

One such film (in color actually) that I rent periodically as a refresher in living splendidly is *Auntie Mame*, the 1958 version with Rosalind Russell. Mame is a fabulous role model for living with excitement and expectation. She tells her nephew, "Your Auntie Mame is going to open doors for you, Patrick, doors you never even dreamed existed"—and she does. She teaches him that "life is a banquet, and most poor suckers are starving to death." Sample this banquet and you'll find yourself filling your plate at the picnic, the potluck, and Thanksgiving dinner with discretion but not deprivation.

This is key to the whole fat business: when you're living fully, you partake of the banquet. That includes food. Food is not the enemy. Using it as a drug, though, expecting it to fill a hole in your soul, is a culprit. Eating food that isn't of the quality you deserve is a bad guy. Too much of a good thing is, well, too much of a good thing; but it doesn't mean that food is out to get you. It just means that you're not sure that something else quite as pleasant as finishing an oversized cookie is on its way to you. By living fully between meals, you make certain that another wonderful occasion or sensation is coming up. When this is the way you live, stopping when you've had enough to eat will get easier—even if it seemed impossible not long ago.

One easy way to live fully is to start saying yes to invitations and opportunities, especially the ones you would have skipped before. Then instigate your own small adventures— taking a class in something you're curious about, trying a new cuisine, inviting an acquaintance out for tea and seeing how many cups it takes to turn you into friends. Eventually, you'll want to insert some grand experiences into the mix: a big trip, a major project, an act of charity that expands your soul.

Some friends and family members may attempt to discourage you because they themselves are afraid. These people need their fears to maintain an orderly worldview. They're like fish in a tank with a clear glass divider. The fish learn to swim in the space available. When the divider is removed, they continue to swim in that same space. A bigger tank—a bigger world—is there for them, but they can't bring themselves to venture into it. People who are frightened by the very thought of living fully do the same thing. That's their business, until they try to get you to do it too.

But what isn't scary can do you in. Snacking doesn't intimidate anybody. Neither does watching TV. Or sitting in a movie with a large drink and so much popcorn that it comes in a tub. Driving to work and parking in the garage doesn't upset any applecarts, but riding your bike and asking for a place to lock it up just might. Suggesting to your boyfriend that you'd like to go to the soup-and-salad place instead of the he-man chuckwagon could be awkward. Hearing your best friend say, "I can't stand you now that you're skinny" (even though she's supposedly joking and you're not "skinny" anyway) could make you feel uncomfortable all afternoon.

The only positive option is to stay on your path and keep your focus. You are committed to living fully. You are going to take care of you, no matter who suggests that you're selfish or full of yourself. Living well will give you the emotional energy you need to fulfill your destiny. Taking care of yourself will give you the physical energy to move beyond fat, broke & lonely and into the life you know you're supposed to be living. Keep at this. Those close to you will either come around or back off, and other people—people who are themselves living fully—will find their way to you.

Take an Action

Take some solid action toward living fully today. Maybe that means putting your morning OJ into a stemmed goblet, or wearing the new outfit you've been saving for something special. This is something special: it's a day of your life. Each one you miss out on means that fat, broke & lonely wins, and that's a shame.

Chapter 15

GOOD FOOD IS A GOOD THING

There is a common belief that good food makes people fat. It can, of course, but in practice far more people are carrying around excess calories from food that wasn't all that great in the first place. I heard an interview with two French women on the topic of Americans. The women said that they liked how friendly we are, and how we're eager to try new things, and how innovative we have historically been as a people. But something perplexed them about us Yanks: "Why are so many Americans fat," one of them wanted to know, "when the food is so bad?" Setting aside any temptation to indulge in transatlantic bickering, you've got to admit that it's a valid question. Very few of us got fat because our hobby was fine dining.

Logically, obesity should be most prevalent among gourmets, chefs, food stylists, and food critics. Although some of them do succumb, my observations suggest that these dyed-in-the-wool foodies are less likely to be significantly overweight than the population in general. In the same way that fashion pros are known for their simple style, people who

genuinely enjoy food dine with discrimination. Serious overeaters may claim to be hopelessly devoted to food as a genre,
but close observation reveals that they turn a few items into
drugs of choice. Mine were soft-serve, trail mix (it's natural,
right?), great whopping chunks of cheese, Planters Peanut
Bars, buttermilk (I know that's warped), and a particular snack
cake whose frosted rectangles courteously came three to a
package instead of the standard two.

Out of the abundance available to me, I picked seven products that, except for the cheese, were cheap as dirt. This from
a person who claimed to feel for food the way Isolde felt for
Tristan! It's embarrassing, but I'm telling you to make a point:
expanding your gastronomic horizons and coming to relish
food as much as you already think you do won't make you fat.
It should help you get thinner.

You can see this even in people who are overweight without being binge eaters. The favorite food for most is familiar
and comforting American fare. Burgers and fries and cherry
pies ... fried chicken and barbecued ribs ... tacos and pizza
(not native to the United States but naturalized for a long
time) ... ice cream and cake ... chips and dip ... sugar-laced
soda (it's the number-one source of calories from sugar, in
fact) and the diet kind that boasts scarcely a calorie of its own
but sure makes you want to eat something.

Again, these people are not, for the most part, poring over
the pages of *Gourmet* and *Cook's Illustrated*. They're not sampling
delectable food and drink from around the world. They aren't
fat because of a hearty lust for the pleasures of the palate, or
even simply because their food is replete with fat and calories
(although it is). They're fat in large part because the food is

uninteresting, inadequate both nutritionally and aesthetically. As a result, they eat more and more of it in a vain attempt to get some satisfaction, but as Mick Jagger will tell you on any oldies station, there is none to be had.

Well, actually there is, but it requires a personal revolution that will affect both the way you eat and the way you live. It calls for a willingness to let go of what seems normal. You can hear it in the words people choose: "We don't have any normal milk—only soy." "Should I buy regular lettuce or the organic kind?" "I'll be in California: I hope I can find something to eat out there that isn't weird." Embrace weird! It's "normal" food that's made us abnormally fat.

Our training in this normal-that-isn't-normal started in childhood. We had different family influences—some of our moms cooked ethnic specialties from scratch, while others nuked diet dinners out of the freezer—but all of us were subject to the influence of the food business. For starters, you've got the fast-food industry cleverly pandering to the hyperactivity its fare may exacerbate by providing compact plastic playgrounds on the premises. The message is, "Go wild, kids. Being civilized is overrated anyway."

And even in sit-down restaurants, take a look at the kids' menus: chicken nuggets, deep-fried by definition; grilled (processed) cheese on white bread; white-flour pasta with meatballs or white-flour macaroni and (processed) cheese; and maybe a kid-sized burger on a white-flour bun with the obligatory fries. These menus are eerily similar in both chains and privately owned eateries around the country. It's as if there's some kid-feeding subcommittee of the Trilateral Commission conspiring to hook yet another generation on sugar, salt, and grease, and train children when they're most teachable that green vegetables, fresh fruits, and whole grains—the fiber-rich foods favored by people who stay trim without dieting—are "yuckeeeee!"

Okay, so you've been brainwashed since you were two. You can reprogram yourself and have fun doing it. Focus on food that grows out of the ground. Explore the produce section of some really great grocery store. Savor a ripe persimmon or an heirloom tomato. Go to a natural foods restaurant. Learn from a book or a class to prepare "spa cuisine," delicious dishes with less reliance on oil, sugar, and salt. Sometimes have an entrée based on legumes (dried beans and peas)—the protein champions of the plant kingdom. Trade in dieting for discovering nature's bounty.

Food that will nourish your body and delight your senses is not the enemy. If some particular item calls to you in such a way that you don't feel safe having it around, don't have it around. Otherwise, compliment God and nature and the chefs and the farmers and the earthworms by choosing foods the planet provides with minimal, if any, interference from manufacturers and marketers. These are beautiful to look at and luscious to taste. They're foods that promise to give you the nutrients you need and that invite you to sit at a table with people you care about, or with yourself and *Frank Sinatra's Greatest Hits*.

Eating—dining—is meant to be a pleasure. So are waking up and going to sleep. Making love and hearing music. Feeling the wind on your face and saluting the sun in yoga class. Talking with a friend and listening to your intuition. Pleasure. Yummy. All of it. Partake and enjoy.

Take an Action

For dinner this very night, have something you want to say grace over, because you are genuinely grateful that it's really this good.

Chapter 16

FIND OUT WHO ISN'T FAT AND DO WHAT THEY DO

After sixty years of dieting, Americans are fatter than ever, and we're exporting fatness around the globe. Instead of coming up with another surefire diet plan, why aren't we looking at those who aren't fat and doing what they do? So who's not fat? Well, there are the chronic dieters and compulsive exercisers, anorexics and many bulimics, and the occasional genetic wonder endowed with an alchemist's ability to metabolize pure lard into muscle and immediately usable energy. Setting aside these out-of-the-ordinary (and the let's-not-go-there) specimens, we can look at who else, as a general rule, avoids being fat and see what they have in common. My listing, alphabetically, consists of:

- *Asians:* Although obesity is creeping into Asia alongside the fast-food franchises, mainland China, the most populous nation on the planet, is still largely free of the problem. Ditto Japan (Sumo wrestlers don't count), Korea, Thailand, and Vietnam. Asia should be the laboratory where we look to see who's doing things right in the kitchen. Think about it: there's this huge continent where billions of people aren't dying early from either starvation or surfeit. They must be doing something right, and that something is the traditional Asian diet, which consists of a basic starch (most often rice, wheat in some regions), lots of fresh vegetables, some fruit, fish, and poultry or pork when it's available and affordable.

- *Athletes and dancers:* I attended an event honoring the writer Toni Morrison. On the program was veteran dancer Bill T. Jones. He had such a deftly sculpted physique (including perfect six-pack abs) that when he came onstage, there was a collective gasp. Turns out he's fifty-four, but he has a body that men half his age would give up premium cable for. With dancers, and athletes who keep moving when they're no longer competing, age is a mere formality. Their vigorous movement creates for them a ninety-ninth percentile body, while the sedentary among us settle for middle-aged spread—although nowadays the spread often starts at puberty and doesn't let up.

- *People in the National Weight Control Registry:* The National Weight Control Registry (www.nwcr.ws) tracks people who have lost more than thirty pounds and kept it off for one year or longer. The majority of registry members report that they avoid gaining back their weight through a diet that is low in overall calories and relatively lower in fat and higher in complex carbohydrates than many dieters now favor. Nearly 80 percent claim to eat breakfast daily. Most also engage in regular exercise.

- *Us, thirty years ago:* Obesity doubled in the United States between 1980 and 2000, in spite of (or, in part, because of) the low-fat diets of the 1980s and the low-carb diets of the 1990s. It snuck in as health clubs blossomed and yoga stopped being confused with yogurt. While some lined up for spinning, cross-training, and Pilates, others were lining up at all-you-can-eat buffets.

  During this time, high-fructose corn syrup, which is cheaper to produce than sugar, its chemical cousin, decreased the cost and increased the size of soft drinks. Vending machines went into schools. We ate out more. Restaurants competed for our business and lured us with larger portions and the salt, sugar, and fat that hook diners in a culinary version of *Reefer Madness*. Fast-food joints, already ubiquitous, achieved restaurant status, and their highly processed, calorific fare started to seem like ordinary food. Weight loss experts traded the conventional wisdom of "Don't eat between meals" for "Eat frequent small meals," translated by anyone at risk for overdoing as "Go ahead and nosh all the time."

  In addition, we went from four TV channels to hundreds, so there was always something to watch. When computers got personal, we sat even more, but without the guilt of the couch potato because this new lethargy sounded so active: we were working, communicating, learning things, making friends, and going shopping. Of course, nothing moved but our fingers, so we got fatter (and broker and lonelier too, but that's another chapter).

- *Vegans:* Vegetarians (people who don't eat meat or fish) are 3 to 20 percent leaner on average than meat-eaters, and vegans (total vegetarians who also avoid dairy products and eggs) have statistically lower BMIs than their more liberally dining cohorts in veggiedom. Nutritional biochemist T. Colin Campbell, Ph.D. (he headed the China Health Study, the largest nutritional investigation ever conducted), states, "Consuming plant-based diets, if in the form of whole foods, will consistently result in a decrease in obesity prevalence."

  A whole-foods, plant-based diet is high in complex carbohydrates (vegetables and whole grains), reasonable in sugars (from fresh and dried fruits), sufficient in the kind of protein that doesn't pack a saturated-fat wallop (the vegetable protein in legumes, soy products, whole grains), and adequate in important fats (nuts, seeds, olive oil, flax). This kind of menu includes crispy salads and crudités; steamed and sautéed veggies; soups and stews and stir-fries; pasta and veggie burgers; baked potatoes, yams, and squash; brown rice, millet, and quinoa; black beans, red beans, chickpeas, and tofu; fruits and berries and everything they served in Eden, apples included.

- *Wild animals:* Unless you're talking about a hibernating species that stores fat as fuel to last the snoozing season, animals in the wild do not get fat. Whether they're carnivores, omnivores, herbivores, or frugivores, creatures do not get fat when they eat the food nature provides for their species. Obviously, humans can function as omnivores, thrive, reproduce, and subdue everybody, but our closest anatomical relatives are the predominantly frugivorous primates. Like them, we have a frugivore's lengthy intestinal tract, grinding molars, and hands suited for picking fruit. When we eat the food suited to our physiology—roots, fruits, leaves, and seeds for the most part—we don't get fat.

  Apparently every animal in existence, with the exception of the one who's supposed to be so smart, knows what to eat and when to stop. Only modern Western humans—and our companion animals, who live more or less the way we do—are at risk for obesity. (Overheard on the Upper East Side: "Winston goes to the dog gym for his workouts. The cat's trainer comes to the apartment." Yes, it does sound like a comment one might hear shortly before the collapse of a civilization, but at least Winston and his feline sibling are staying in shape.)

There is a theme in these bullet points: staying at a healthy body size doesn't have to be a big deal. It needn't be complicated, torturous, or harrowing. In the vast majority of cases, it does not require a rigid diet, drugs or surgery, an in-depth understanding of nutrition, or a trainer whose other jobs are drill sergeant and dominatrix.

If you want to stop being fat or stop worrying about getting fat, eat real food, predominantly from the plant kingdom. If you don't know what "real food, predominantly from the plant kingdom" is or how to fix it, go to the library or bookstore and look through vegetarian and natural foods cookbooks. (I've included my faves in the bibliography.) Spend an hour in a well-stocked health food store. Befriend the produce guy at your supermarket. Go to the farmers' market and talk to farmers. Ask the people who grow it what to do with kale (hack off the tough stems and steam the leaves with a little olive oil and a lot of garlic) or acorn squash (cut it in half, scoop out the seeds, lightly brush with olive oil, drizzle with agave nectar—a honeylike natural sweetener that's low on the Glycemic Index—and bake until tender).

Do a fridge-and-cupboard revamp by getting the very sweet, very salty, highly processed foods out of your kitchen. When you go out, steer clear of fast food: care enough about yourself to eat in a place that has dishes and a waitstaff. Drink water (still or sparkling) or iced tea or half-juice/half-seltzer instead of soda. When you're having a treat, go for tall instead of *venti*, one scoop instead of three. Unless your doctor says you must do otherwise, eat breakfast, lunch, and dinner, and spend your time *living* instead of snacking in between.

Make regular exercise a part of your day and fit in incidental exercise too—walking where you're going, climbing stairs, doing the labor of maintaining yourself. Find ways to enjoy activity: you can take tango lessons, hike in the woods, join a cycling group, learn to Rollerblade. You may want to think of this as recreation rather than exercise. Otherwise, it could be like an office party: you're supposed to be having a great good time, but you're really still at work.

Take an Action

Adopt as your own today one habit borrowed from those who are not fat. Keep at this one thing until it's yours for keeps. When you have it down, make other small changes—even one at a time if that's what it takes to get them to stick.

Chapter 17

WHEN IN DOUBT, USE THE MAP (MODERATION, ACTIVITY, PERSISTENCE)

People who aren't fat engage in certain simple disciplines:

1. They're moderate in what they consume.

2. They lead physically active lives.

3. They're persistent in doing what's necessary to keep themselves in check and in shape.

Millions of men and women do this unconsciously. It's the way they were brought up, the way they've always been. Others, a goodly number of whom were once fat, practice moderation, activity, and persistence until these seem normal, or even if they never quite seem normal. Moderation, Activity, and Persistence "map" the way out of fat. (They can help with broke and lonely, too, since once you develop discipline, it's transferable to other areas of life.)

Moderation: Moderation is knowing when enough is enough. In relation to food, it's stopping just before you think you're full because in a land of plenty it's easy to mistake *stuffed* for *full.* Do not be fooled: those heartburn and indigestion commercials air in primetime because we don't know when to stop. If you're unsure what moderation looks like, consult this brief list of examples:

- A great big salad (since raw vegetables are mostly water, a salad can look huge and be moderate as long as you keep the dressing down to two tablespoons).

- A mid-sized plate of pasta (that's what they serve at an upscale Italian restaurant where portions are about half that of a typical bargain spot).

- The whole serving of brown rice at a Chinese restaurant and half the entrée (the rice is a fat-free, fiber-rich filler food; General Tso's whatever is going to be rich and oily. If you opt for a steamed entrée, you can eat more of it and still be moderate).

- A piece of meat (if you eat meat) is moderate when it's the size of a deck of cards.

- Two envelopes of instant oatmeal (one is a "serving," but two are still moderate and not unreasonable if you're hungry in the morning).

- Four ounces—that's half a *cup*, not half of a Lord-knows-how-much-this-thing-holds mug—of orange juice (if you squeeze it yourself, you'll understand how many oranges it takes to make a wee glassful).

- Half a restaurant dessert, or even a three- or four-way split (a little sweetness can be nice after a meal; a whole dessert is a sugar shock nobody needs).

- One standard-sized dinner plate of the various components that make up dinner, with some plate showing around the edges. No second helpings. (If you eat slowly, you'll give your brain the twenty minutes it needs to get the message that you've been fed.)

- One nutrition bar that actually has nutrition in it. I'm sold on the LUNA bar, but there are several good brands out there. For breakfast (when there really is no time for breakfast), or something sweet at the end of a meal, or an afternoon snack (when you know you won't be having dinner until after the movie), choose a bar that's under 200 calories; steers clear of refined sugar, high fructose corn syrup, and hydrogenated oils; and has a respectable amount of protein (7 to 10 grams).

- A vintage bottle of soda. If you drink soda at all (which I discourage on principle: it does nothing for you and you're worth better), buy those cute little bottles modeled on the six- and eight-ounce sizes of yesteryear —you know, back when people weren't fat.

Activity: Most of us learned in first grade that all life is either animal, vegetable, or mineral. The latter two don't move. Animals, human and the other kinds, are so named because we're *animate*. Accept it: you are neither a begonia nor a boulder; you're supposed to be moving.

The simple discipline of activity recognizes that, unless you're a longshoreman or otherwise work at a job that involves rigorous and sustained use of your musculature, you have to exercise.

Do it in the morning even if you hate morning; that way you know it's done. (And if you exercise before breakfast you'll get through your glycogen reserves in about five minutes instead of twenty, so you'll be burning fat more quickly.) If you're past forty, get your doctor's permission; then exercise to the point of serious sweat a minimum of three days a week. Ideally, you'll work up to exercising every day of the week but one. This routine might look like: thirty minutes of cardio (running, dancing, the treadmill, energetic walking) and ten minutes of stretching four days a week, and two days of weight-training, each session about forty minutes long and covering both upper and lower body. (Schedule at least one day, even two, between your workouts with weights.)

If you're ill, lay off until you're well, and then get back as if you were reporting to a probation officer. If you're injured, exercise the parts of yourself that aren't. And slip in additional activity every chance you get. Park in the farthest spot instead of the nearest. Drive a stick shift. Climb the stairs. Walk the dog. Refuse to move to a block that doesn't have sidewalks.

Persistence: Persistence is mandatory. You don't eat well once and figure you've done that, or take a six-week jazz dance course and check "exercise" off your lifetime to-do list. If you are persistent, you refuse to take a vacation from taking care of yourself, even if you are on vacation. You don't let your inability to be perfect keep you from being pretty darned good. With persistence, a setback is a mere speed bump; without it, you're looking at a four-car pileup.

This is for life. This is life. Every day, treat yourself like someone worth nurturing and preserving. Every day, stay vigilant to the excuses that would take you back to the old, fat-attracting way of doing things. And every single day invite, expect, and allow in help from your Higher Power. It's never out of reach but you have to renew the connection on a daily basis.

Persistence is necessary because your default mechanism may have been set a long time ago at either "fat" or "fear of fat." Letting things slide can mean sliding back. However—and this is big—persistence is not paranoia or obsession with your diet and exercise habits. If you find yourself so concerned about these that you're missing out on life, something's not right. Are you getting your quiet time (chapter 9) every morning? Are there supportive people around you? Are you sleeping enough? And dealing with hurts and slights and disappointments before they morph into monsters? If so, there's nothing to keep you from persisting in the way of freedom. Don't be afraid. You might choose to pass on the cocktails or the dessert, but you never have to miss the party.

Take an Action

Look at your relationship with your body today and ascertain which would benefit you more right now: a little more moderation or a little more activity. Commit to that. Because moderation and activity enjoy each other's company, sticking with one means that you'll be incorporating both and getting persistence in the bargain.

Chapter 18

I KNOW THIS MUCH IS TRUE

Your life is your life and you'll find your way by finding your way. I have, however, managed to avoid being fat for, gosh, twenty-three years now, and as a result there are some truths I hold as sacrosanct. You're welcome to take any of these that work for you. File the others away somewhere; one or two that just seem dumb right now could look a lot better later.

These things I know to be true:

- *Mornings are for ME: Meditation and Exercise.* Tending to "me" in the morning sets me up for my day and whatever demands it makes, and it can do the same for you.

- *Self-care is mandatory.* If you need lunch and your husband wants to keep driving or sightseeing or mowing the lawn, demand your right to have lunch. If having cookies in the cupboard drives you nuts but your kids want them, give them the life lesson that nobody gets what they want all the time. *You count.* If you act as if you don't, you'll have to get really large just to prove you're here.

- *Sleep is important.* If you get enough sleep, you'll awaken early and feel refreshed. Exercising when you're overtired predisposes a body to injury, and sleep deprivation can lead to a god-awful sugar craving. Sure, there are some legitimate reasons for staying out late, and when you have one, live a little. When you don't, go for healthy, wealthy, and wise.

- *Without enough water, you'll feel hungry.* Being even a little dehydrated can throw your thirst mechanism out of whack. Your dried-up brain is apt to cry for glucose (sugar) when you really need water.

- *Skipping breakfast is asking for trouble.* You've just been on a ten- or twelve- or fourteen-hour fast. If you're not feeling hungry yet, you don't have to eat a big breakfast; some people do fine on a couple of pieces of fruit. Most of us fare better with something more substantial. There's a lot of staying power in a little protein teamed with a complex carbohydrate. Experiment. Just don't go out into the world without some fuel.

- *Grazing is for cattle.* I know, I know, experts are chanting, "Graaaaze," like some magical mantra, but unless you have a medical condition that requires it, grazing is just binging stretched out. Eat three times a day and

develop the courage, grace, and poise to keep food out
of your mouth the rest of the time.

- *Dieting makes people fat.* The highway that runs by Diet
  Town has only two exits: Deprivation and Indulgence.
  The locals call them "on" and "off." Both are extreme
  and counterproductive. Drive on to Sanityville, where
  there's nothing to fall off of. If you've dieted for a long
  time, Sanityville will resemble a mirage, like "Toto, I
  have a feeling we're not in Kansas anymore," if Kansas
  is the only place you've ever been. Persist. In time you'll
  feel right at home.

- *Drugs and alcohol can interfere.* Drugs, even when they're
  prescribed or you buy them over a common counter to
  treat a common cold, may affect your appetite and your
  ability to easily refrain from overeating. Even caffeine,
  an appetite suppressant in the short run, can make you
  want to consume a food court once it wears off.
  Alcohol has calories of its own to consider, and if
  drinking puts you in a throw-caution-to-the-wind frame
  of mind, this may be something for you to look at.

- *Junky feelings lead to junky food.* Envy. Resentment.
  Coveting thy neighbor's ass. Wanting somebody else's
  advantages because there don't seem to be enough
  slated for you. I once didn't binge for *four years*, got
  angry and jealous at a friend, and started a six-month
  bacchanal with a bag of—I'm not kidding—prunes. No
  irritating person and no irritating situation is worth
  eating over. Maybe a walk or some deep breathing

would help. You might need to call someone and talk it out. Whatever it takes, protect yourself from any emotions that could lead to layer cake—or if you're really far gone, prunes.

- *Your Higher Power is interested in everything that interests you.* This includes an obsession with cheese puffs and white-chocolate bunnies. Expecting the loving Force inside you to change your attitude toward food and the way you see your body is not foolhardy, or asking too much, or abandoning personal responsibility. You expect God (or something like God) to keep the earth rotating and do the rest of the cosmic housekeeping. Why not get some assistance from the top when you want to say "marinara" and you sense "Alfredo" about to come out?

Some of what I know is true I've learned from other people. Experience has taught me the rest. As you go forward committed to your own well-being, you'll unearth more and more that you know to be true. Trust it, even if it's only today's truth and tomorrow might reveal something else. It's all any of us has to go on.

You see, I could tell you that fat will never darken your door (or widen your hips) if you do precisely what I do and live precisely as I live. Someone who read a book I wrote about overcoming overeating, *Fit from Within*, e-mailed me: "You'd be famous like Atkins if you just didn't give people so much autonomy." But without autonomy, you're an automaton.

By this time you have a pretty good idea about what I think and what I do. I eat three times a day as a general rule. I'm a vegetarian and pretty close to vegan. (I believe it's a healthy way to eat, but mostly I do it because I've been to a slaughterhouse and a factory egg farm, and I don't want to be part of what goes on in those places.) I believe in eating whole foods, minimally tampered with, organic when possible. Discovering new foods and exotic cuisines is fun for me, and I've learned that "discovering" and "binging" are light-years apart. I don't do a lot of pre-maneuvering around food, and I rarely pack a lunch or tote a cooler. That would put me back in the food business from which I've long since retired. I figure that when mealtime comes, there will be some acceptable food wherever I am. I haven't gone hungry yet. I don't stress or obsess about food; but if some carton of carryout in the fridge is on my mind more than it ought to be, I toss it.

I've never liked exercise, but I make sure it gets done, and afterward I like it well enough. Right now, I do weights and the treadmill at the gym two or three times a week; the other mornings I walk with my husband to Central Park, where we crawl over the rock outcroppings and call it rock-climbing.

I could abandon these exercise and eating practices in a Manhattan minute if my attitude weren't in the right place, but I have friends who won't let me off the hook and who model for me the kind of behavior I strive to practice. Left to my own devices, I would without question be lying on a couch, watching TV, slurping something cold and creamy, and wondering why I had no life. Letting God, as I see God, be in charge today means that I'm not left to my own devices.

That's me. I'm not famous like Atkins, but I know this much is true. Take what you like. Then make your own way.

Take an Action

Write an inventory of what you know is true for yourself—regarding food, exercise, and body image, but in other areas, too, if your pen wants to go there. Read over the list a few times and give it some thought. Act on what you know is true.

Chapter 19

ONE OTHER PERSON HAS TO BE IN ON THIS

People sometimes overeat in groups—witness Thanksgiving—but there is no social binging. If you want to eat something you're ashamed of, you'll do it by yourself. This is why it's essential to have people, or at least one person, with you on the road to freedom. He, she, or they become your witness(es). You're far more likely to keep at a new way of living when at least one other breathing being has seen where you've come from and will tell you straight if you're rationalizing or entering dangerous territory.

Not just any old *homo sapiens* will do. It's patently loony to share your food problems with your husband, the girls at the office, or even your very best friend if these people don't get it. Turn to a support group, face-to-face or online, or a friend you believe to be as committed to transforming her life as you are to transforming yours.

My friend Sherry is one of those for me. She'll tell anybody: "I don't drink." "I don't eat sugar." "I don't eat between meals." And she doesn't. Sherry and I are "action partners." This means that she's committed to my best life and I am to hers. For outgrowing the baby fat that may have been with you for thirty years, or for revolutionizing your life in other ways, this kind of partnership can be a godsend. It calls for two imperfect but committed people who are willing to be honest with themselves and each other.

For action-partnering to work—whether for fat, broke, lonely, or something else—you need to be in contact regularly and often. Meeting every day by phone and once a week in person is ideal. Voice mail is okay, and text-messaging and e-mail are better than not making contact, but don't use them as digital muumuus you can hide inside. It's easier to lie when you don't have body language or at least vocal intonations to reveal what's really going on. And when you do talk, don't go on at length. Chitchat is open-ended; getting two lives on track for a day takes about ten minutes.

Your action partner is not your therapist, and she's not being paid to listen to you kvetch. Of course you can share what's happening right now and what you're afraid of, but venting (short-form, please) needs to be a prelude to action. Say what needs to be said and then get out and build the life you claim to want more than anything.

One of the most useful practices in which you can engage with your action partner is *parenthesizing*—putting invisible parentheses around an action by telling the other person what you plan to do and calling her back after you've done it. This works particularly well when you're faced with a task that's difficult or intimidating or when there's something you have to do and you just plain don't wanna. For example, I might call Sherry and say: "My cold lasted three days, but I haven't been to the gym for four." And she'll tell me: "Get your sneakers on and get over there *now*. Call me when you're in the door, and call again after you've worked out." Of course I do it: I'm all of a sudden accountable to somebody.

Action partners are co-mentors. You don't have to have all the answers, but you can share your wisdom with your friend and draw on hers. If you're in a position of authority in your work, having an action partner is a distinct relief. This is one place where the buck doesn't stop with you. Doubts and uncertainties are allowed. And you don't have to relinquish your self-esteem or your place in the world to enjoy this lightening of your load.

When you're someone's action partner, you're inspired to make better choices. Another human being is in on them now. On the one hand, it's a responsibility: someone is counting on you. On the other, you're buoyed up because you don't have to face personal challenges and difficulties on your own. Besides, if you really screw up, you'll have to tell her. (Or him—guys should action-partner guys, and women should action-partner women.)

In addition to your action partner, have other people around you who are living conscious, positive lives (see chapter 43, "Put Together Your Dream Team"). It's like when you were a teenager and your mom wanted you to befriend the kids who'd be "good influences." At any age, you'll never regret hanging out with people you have to stretch to keep up with. As much as we like to think that we're masters of our fate and captains of our souls (and maybe even of the *Starship Enterprise*), we tend to act like the people around us. Remember: we're tribal creatures. We feel safe when we do what other members of our tribe do. Therefore, it's a bright idea to add to your tribe people who eat healthfully, stay fit, and have a spiritual life. You'll meet them at the gym and the yoga studio and in clubs and classes where people who are interested in enlightened living go. You will find them when you expect to find them: put out the intention and know that these people are heading your way.

I think one of the reasons the recidivism rate for overeating is so high—greater than for reformed heroin addicts, I've read—is that losing weight has traditionally been a solitary undertaking. The little extra here, the hidden pastry there, creeps back in a similarly solitary fashion. People who join weight loss groups do better. Those who opt for camaraderie and a change that starts on the inside and moves on out do the best. When you have a friend who cares enough to tell you when you're full of it, you have a really good chance. If she'll come down to the Häagen-Dazs and drag you out of there before they can get the cherry on your sundae, you're in good hands.

Take an Action

Get an action partner. If you have an eating problem, find someone who's overcoming an eating problem of her own and has a philosophy similar to yours. If you just want to lose a few inches and be more regular with exercise, find someone with comparable objectives. If you're only reading this to get to the part about "broke" or "lonely," get yourself an action partner who has goals similar to yours. Talk every day or almost every day. Be as honest as you've ever been.

Chapter 20

WITH A HIGHER POWER, WILLPOWER IS SO LAST SEASON

You probably don't need a single piece of information about diet and exercise beyond what you already have. Women's magazines are full of it, as are newspapers, newscasts and TV specials, and the click-on headlines you get when you retrieve your e-mail. The gap is between knowing and doing. To close it, we've depended on willpower, but after repeated wounding in the diet wars, chances are your willpower is shot. No problem. *There is a power inside you that leads to right decisions, even in areas as ordinary as your food choices and getting to the gym.* When you're tuned in to the strength inside that doesn't come from your ego, you shift from half-power to Higher Power. Everything is different after that.

Know that within you at this moment and every moment you live is an Intelligence that is invested in your well-being, your happiness, your growth, and your shining at maximum wattage. When your communication with this Intelligence is unimpeded, your will aligns with that will, and you want what's good for you in the myriad ways that "good for you" can play out.

This connection to a Higher Power is essential because habit digs deep grooves in a life. Trying to plug these pits yourself is a trial of mythical proportions. With a Higher Power, and your participation of course, they fill in and smooth over. The surest way to make the tiny, crucial shift from ego-powered to Higher-Powered living is to decide that that's your choice and then to live your life based on that decision. This way of living, as Rudolph Nureyev said of ballet, "never becomes easy, but it does become possible." To the best of my knowledge, the following summarizes a viable way to acquire and nurture a spiritual life for anyone who has at times sought God in a convenience store:

- *Give up going it alone.* Allow for a God that loves you even more than you love baked goods. And as we discussed in the previous chapter, get yourself some buddies who are acquainted with both a Higher Power and chocolate-chip cookies.

- *Entertain the possibility* (if possibility is as far as you can go) *that there is a force for good in your life* that doesn't want you either stuffed and remorseful or dieting and irritated as hell.

- *Pretend that this is true until you believe it.* When you're at a restaurant and you're craving the entire deep-fried section, or when the office clock says 3:00 and you know that 5:00 will never come without a snack, call on your Higher Power. Go to the ladies' room (guys: the other one), stand in the stall, and say, "Okay, God, things don't look great at this moment, but I'm trusting. I expect you to come through." If you're at that restaurant, go back and order what is, *in your opinion,* the loveliest, healthiest, most delicious, most appropriate meal on the menu (or even not on the menu: you can ask for a little innovation from the kitchen). If you're at work, go back to your desk and feign interest. This too shall pass.

- *Stop watching your weight and just wait.* Waiting—from dinner to bedtime, or for your friend to finish that muffin the size of a UFO—means that you're trusting that you won't die or go crazy or do a *Jaws*-like attack on a Taco Bell. You just wait. Time passes. Peace shows up. Life fills in the blanks, and you realize you've been taken care of.

- *Pray a new way.* Although every sincere prayer has merit, begging and pleading presumes that you can convince the organizing, orchestrating Energy of life to change course. But since God already wants the best for you, an alternative method of prayer is to align your thoughts with God's thoughts as you're able to conceive of them. Therefore, if you're not getting very far with "Keep me from slivering through this entire pan of lasagna and I'll be good forever," you might try "Through the power of God within me, I am satisfied and content."

- *Start acting like the Light that's inside you.* Networking experts will tell you that to bond with a new acquaintance, it helps if your clothing, mannerisms, and references are somewhat like his. To get better acquainted with the Light within, be more like it. This Light is generous and expansive. It's available for everyone. Its purpose is to dispel darkness. You can, in your own world and in your own way, do that too.

- *Let Spirit express through your body as well as your soul.* We're so split in Western culture—thoughts versus feelings, the way things are versus the way they could be, body versus spirit. But the body reflects the spirit. When you're at peace inside, you'll take fine care of your outsides—and you'll have a lovely sparkle about you too: kind of like being in love but without having to worry if he's ready to commit.

- *Keep things simple.* One meal at a time. One experience of fitting-room humility at a time. One spinning class completed. One snub overlooked. One piece of toast left on the plate. One day lived reasonably well considering that perfection is not native to this region.

- *Be so grateful it's hokey.* Gratitude is as filling as pancakes. As you go through your day, be grateful for every good thing you see and smell and taste and experience. Be grateful for the sun and the rain, your second-best friend and your favorite turtleneck and that you have TiVo.

- *Allow for happiness, contentment, and satisfaction.* These are not nearly as sexy as angst and ambition. Some see happiness, contentment, and satisfaction as evidence of being too out of the loop to understand how bad things really are and how much there is to do. Granted, there is plenty to do. You'll do it more effectively when you're happy, content, and—for this twenty-four-hour period—satisfied. You'll still work and plan and build a better life and a better world. You just won't need to do it with a cellophane-wrapped sidekick.

I wish I could give all this to you—just hand it over like the car keys or five bucks. But you have to discover it yourself. And when you do, it will be yours to keep. That's when fat and dieting and related nemeses become memories and freedom shows up as a gift, there to open every morning.

Take an Action

Live today as if a Power exists in the universe and in yourself that wants only the best for you. A Love for you that doesn't waver, even when your regard for yourself slips a notch or two or ten. A Light that is there to lead you to the life that's been calling you all along. Remind yourself of this on the hour or the half-hour. Do the things today that someone aware of this Power, this Love, and this Light would do.

Part Three

BREAKING UP WITH BROKE

*Abundance—financial and otherwise—is normal,
natural, and right. You attract it by thinking, speaking,
and living abundantly.*

Things works properly when everyone has enough. You too.
You are supposed to have sufficient resources to support
the lifestyle that supports your destiny. Although most people
have to work for money, no one should have to anguish over
it. And yet we do.

We crave objects and possessions that will make us appear
richer or more in the know. We stay at jobs we can't stand to
pay for symbols of our coolness. When our salary can't cover
them all, the purveyors of plastic come to our temporary aid.
Since saving is a disconcerting prospect ("That's my money—
I should be able to spend it"), many of us don't have a calam-
ity cushion. One illness or a sustained period of unemployment
can spell disaster.

When the situation is sufficiently grave, we might go on a
crash diet, this time with money. We put the credit cards in a

drawer and bring lunch in a bag. We skip "unnecessaries" like dental work and an oil change. Before you know it, the filling becomes a crown, the engine goes on strike, and we're so darned sick of pauperism that we say yes to the next credit card offer and, in typical post-diet fashion, go nuts.

And yet abundance is normal, natural, and right. The first step in attracting it is to shut out the lies: "More is always better," "You're not deserving," and "Everybody owes money. It's no big deal." The next move is to think, speak, and live abundantly, both by using dollars-and-cents good sense in your quotidian affairs and by learning and applying the spiritual principles that pertain to money, success, and fulfillment. These will open you to the richness of the universe and to sweet, simple pleasures that don't have to cost a dime.

Chapter 21

IT WASN'T IN THE FRIDGE, AND IT'S NOT AT THE MALL

I was toying with writing a whole book on this subject. My working title was *It's Not About the Money*, but I gave that title to a financial services guy since I figured he had a platform in the world of money. I, on the other hand, have a platform in the world of broke.

You see, one kind of filler behavior fuels another. When I was eating like there was no tomorrow, I also ate my way through an editorial assistant's salary and was reduced, once or twice, to selling postage stamps on the bus to get the few quarters I was short on for the ride. Even without overeating, however, I've at times been tempted by the allure of romanticized poverty. For a while there was "I'm a poor single mother" (which I was, but gosh, the more I reiterated that fact, the nicer and more sympathetic people got). Another fallback was "I'm an artist. We're supposed to be starving. Here's to *la vie bohème!*" That one was fun because you can get really fly stuff at a Salvation Army store, and besides, using old orange crates for bookshelves is so shabby-chic.

The problem with being broke, though, whether it's the serious wolf-at-the-door kind or just continual, coupon-clipping worry, is that the longer you're in it, the more normal it feels. It can get so comfortable, in fact, that it can lead to sabotaging perfectly good prosperity when it's trying to get to you. You might, for instance, quit a job before there's another in the offing, or make a purchase or take a trip that causes you to have to white-knuckle it for three months. It can get to the point where you can feel that, on a very personal level, you and money have irreconcilable differences.

Looking at it from the macro point of view, i.e., society as a whole, I'd say that when it comes to money our society is, let's see, goofy. Look at us. The United States is supposedly the richest country on earth, and yet we're four commas in debt. For an individual, spending money that isn't yours is no longer considered a shameful last resort, it's the accepted way to buy your kids' school clothes and take a friend to dinner. A while back, I was in line at a large hardware store, got out cash for my purchase, and the clerk said, "You don't see much of that anymore." Is this the brave new world? You betcha.

One fundamental cause of both feeling broke and being broke is easy credit. A few years ago, the postman brought one of those "You have been approved!" letters from a major credit card company addressed to Aspen Moran. She's part chocolate Lab and part generic bird dog, but somebody must have thought she could come up with the monthly minimums. At least dogs don't reach adulthood with $80,000 in student loans for a degree that is more and more necessary and less and less valuable. It's no wonder a lot of humans feel broke: they've been in the hole since they took their SATs.

Moreover, as with the fat issue, our culture gives confounding messages about money. Old episodes of *Friends* imply that you can rent a giant apartment in Greenwich Village while working as a massage therapist or barista. Best-sellers swear that we're all living next to millionaires. Adult ed catalogs promise that a yacht and polo ponies are in your future if you just invest in real estate, fix the place up, rent it out, sell it off, and do it again. The message comes across as, "This is so easy, loser, why aren't you doing it?"

It's no wonder a great many of us suffer monetary anxiety expressed as overspending, underearning, unsustainable deprivation (financial anorexia), and unsecured debts to juggle like tennis balls. People without obvious money troubles can feel broke, too, when they've "bought too much house" or the car turns out to be a lemon in jeep's clothing.

At the root of it all is the invisible enemy: emptiness. "There isn't enough ... I can't make enough ... I will never be enough." And the messages aren't just in your head: they're coming at you from marketers who imply that without buying their products and services you'll be old, ugly, smelly, stupid, unquestionably out of touch, and possibly in danger of losing life, limb, and love. Advertisers are well aware that presenting the positive qualities of the widget in question is far less effective than scaring the pants off you with the physical, social, or financial disaster sure to ensue if you don't buy what they're selling. This gets us to acquire a lot of stuff, but nobody has a big enough credit line to buy it all, so we're carrying around

messages of personal deficiency in every area in which we've
done insufficient palliative purchasing.

The empty pit in your psyche that says, "There's never
going to be enough money; that's why the earth brought
forth MasterCard," suggests that since everything else is for
sale, the answer to having a canyon inside must have a price
too. It has to be simply a matter of procuring enough
money—and that's only a stock tip, lottery ticket, or rich guy
away. But if the elixir of life, the filler of emptiness, were
indeed in the Neiman Marcus catalog, the very rich would
buy it and they'd all be very happy. There would be no con-
voluted divorces, no drug-crazed parties, no attempted sui-
cides in the Hills of Beverly. But there are. That's because the
peace that makes life livable is beyond price: *it wasn't in the
fridge, and it's not at the mall.*

This doesn't mean that the answer is a two-piece loincloth
and a begging bowl. It is, rather, to fill the inner void with
inner qualities—trust, purpose, love—and live in a way that
enriches all concerned. Certainly you should have plenty of
money. Money can be used to end suffering and open minds.
That's why *you* ought to have it instead of some selfish, close-
minded person. You need total lucidity on this, however: it's
the intangibles that fill you up. Although wealth is not a re-
quirement for doing good in the world, money can free you
to be of greater use. And when you're of use, you get more
intangibles.

Take an Action

Get out a notebook and pen and assess your relationship with money. How do you two get along? Where are the problem areas? What lies about money have you bought into? What do you want the truth of your financial life to be?

Chapter 22

THE TWELVE STOPS

Ours is a get-ahead culture, and we're always ready to start something that could improve our situation. We're not as thrilled about stopping what caused the trouble in the first place. If finances are sufficiently problematic that "broke" was what attracted you to this book, you need to stop what you're doing and make a serious turnaround. Here are some guidelines. They seem harsh, but they cut to the chase. I think of them as the Twelve Stops:

1. *Stop expecting the world to owe you a living.* Publishers Clearinghouse is a pretty iffy bet. Unless you are truly disabled (and lots of disabled people still support themselves) or you have children who would otherwise suffer, stop asking for exceptions, extensions, a reduced fee, or a sliding scale. Pay your way. When you do, you'll feel wealthy and that will help you attract wealth. If you choose instead not to expend the funds in the first place, fine: you've saved money and your self-respect.

2. *Stop blaming.* Stop blaming Mom who was a compulsive spender and Dad who was a compulsive hoarder and Grandma who didn't put you in the will. They owed you for eighteen years. Period. If you're over eighteen, they're sprung. Free and clear. Fair? Maybe not, but it's the way things work.

3. *Stop spending money that isn't yours.* If you're not using cash (or a check or debit card for an account that actually has money in it), you're borrowing at best, and if you won't be paying the bill in full at the end of the month, you are, for now anyway, stealing. In other words, get rid of those debt cards (not debit: *debt*) that are keeping you from carrying a stylish, slender billfold and attaining financial freedom.

4. *Stop making excuses.* Be willing to do whatever is required to stay out of hock. This could mean working for a time at a job that's "beneath you"—if the paycheck doesn't bounce, the job isn't beneath you. "Whatever is required" could also require, for now, giving up your designer haircutter, cleaning your own house, and bathing your own dog.

5. *Stop looking for a bailout.* Instead, get assistance for your own efforts. Many debt consolidation companies are above reproach and can act as a lifeline for pulling you out of the hole. However, research them carefully. If what they're offering sounds painless, the pain might come when you find out you've been had. The nonprofit volunteer organization Debtors Anonymous

(www.debtorsanonymous.org) can help you help
yourself get out of debt and grow up, whatever your
age. They'll teach you how to be responsible and still
put your own needs first. "Underearners," even those
who have little or no debt but can't seem to break
through the cash ceiling, are welcome at DA too.

6. *Stop, ladies, searching for Mr. Right with the big wallet.* These
days a lot of guys are searching for Ms. Right with a big
purse. When an online dating profile says "financially
secure," that means, when it's true, that this person can
take care of himself or herself. It doesn't mean he or she
wants to take care of you—not to mention your ailing
mother, the two kids from your former marriage, and
the loans you incurred getting your degree in pre-
Jacobean poetry.

7. *Stop vaporizing money.* If yours seems to disappear, write
down what you spend until you know exactly where it
goes. Then make changes you can live with. They don't
all have to be agonizing. If you can get a better deal on
car insurance or lawn care or lower interest rates on
your old debt, you'll end up with more discretionary
money.

8. *Stop letting other people decide your fiscal priorities.* It's been
estimated that *every day* the average American is
exposed to three thousand marketing messages— and
each one is someone trying to influence our fiscal
priorities. Don't let them. You know that song "You and
Me Against the World"? Sing it to your money. You

guys have to be a team and stand strong. Even financial
writers shouldn't make your spending choices. If you
listen to them, you'd never have another latté, which is
just too sacrificial if you're one who looks forward all
week to premium foam and the Sunday crossword.

9.   *Stop shopping as a hobby.* Whether in the stores, online,
     through catalogs, or on TV, retail therapy heals only
     those with something to sell. I know it's fun to look at
     pretty things, and I'm not suggesting that you deny
     yourself anything that you need or even want, if you
     can pay for it. Recreational shopping is, however, the
     shortest distance between two points: you and broke.

10. *Stop collecting crap.* Excuse the vernacular, but you know
     you've got some. We all do. The point is to refrain from
     surrounding yourself with the cheap and the garish.
     You'll feel more prosperous if you have fewer things but
     what you have is lovely. Quality needn't cost a lot. You
     can find it in a piece of original art, even from a flea
     market, or in a well-made jacket, whether from Saks
     Fifth Avenue or the consignment store on Main Street.

11. *Stop talking poor.* "I never have any money." "For what
     they pay at this place, I'll be working when I'm ninety."
     "That's too rich for my blood." Yada, yada. Here's an
     adage for you: "Whine not, want not." In other words,
     live within your means and put a lid on it.

12. *Stop badmouthing the rich.* Face it: we want to be rich so we
     talk about how frivolous and undeserving those who
     are can be—the cars they don't even drive, the servants

they underpay, that last nip/tuck that crossed the line. Let it rest. If having money is all that bad, your subconscious will do everything possible to keep you from such a terrible fate.

The Twelve Stops will plug the leaks. From there you can start to build your financial stability, develop a prosperity consciousness, and create a richer life.

Take an Action

Of the Twelve Stops, select the one that most appeals to you and the one that irritates you more than any of the others. Put these two into practice immediately.

Chapter 23

MAYBE BORING
BUT NEVER BROKE

I was a junior in high school when I saw a touring production of *The Fantasticks*. When the young heroine cried out, "Please, God, don't let me be normal!" I tingled in agreement in the mezzanine. I wasn't about to be one of those everyday people with a mortgage and a paycheck and insurance for everything. I was too intelligent, too creative, too interesting. And for the next twenty-five years I continued to be intelligent, creative, interesting—and often close to broke.

I didn't even think much about it. There was always enough somehow, and I was proud that I lived such a colorful life on so little green. I had no reserves to speak of, but I figured I didn't need them since I'd one day inherit money from my dad. Well, I didn't. It was a tale of almost Springer-esque sleaze. When I was living on the other side of the country, an unscrupulous woman married my elderly father and, with the aid of her boyfriend (I told you it was sleazy), changed the will, put all my father's assets into joint accounts, and got everything. She was a dreadful person, but in one way she did me a service in spite of herself. If I'd inherited money at forty, I'd have stayed fourteen financially for the rest of my life.

Realizing that *heiress* was never going in the occupation space on my Form 1040, I woke from my fiscal slumber and found out that, in the same way that fat had lost its "overwhelming" status a decade before, broke was not an immutable force that was out to get me. I didn't have money because I hadn't really wanted it. I'd picked up somewhere that financial stability would make me boring and fence me in. Armed with this rationalization, I hadn't had to be fully responsible for myself.

When the student is ready to get her act together, teachers do appear. I found a book called *Your Money or Your Life* by Joe Dominguez and Vicki Robin, about achieving financial independence and then devoting your energies to improving life on earth. A group of women met at my place every Tuesday night to study it.

Concurrently, I enrolled in a prosperity class at a local church and learned about the inner side of abundance. When I wasn't making as much progress as the other people in the class, the instructor told me that I needed to clear the way in a practical, bottom-line sense before I'd be ready for spiritual principles. When he told me to read *How to Get Out of Debt, Stay Out of Debt, and Live Prosperously* by Jerrold Mundis, I was ticked off. I told him I wasn't in debt—well, you know, not like *most people*. He said, "I know. Read it anyway." I did. It filled in more missing pieces.

The information in these books and classes and others that followed coalesced for me into a body of knowledge, a financial philosophy of life. It took some time—I rebel against change, and that's how I know you probably do too—but eventually I came to see that there are ironclad ways to avoid ever being broke. They are:

- *Live on a cash economy.* This means pay as you go. "Neither a borrower nor a lender be." No loans unless they're secured, i.e., backed up by collateral. (A house is collateral for the bank; a diamond ring is collateral for a pawn shop.) No credit card unless you pay it off easily and consistently every month or, if you're a credit junkie, no credit card at all (see chapter 24).

- *Deal with debt by not making any more of it.* Take care of what's there by (1) finding a way to cut the interest, and (2) paying off the rest *slowly* so there's enough money left for a decent life starting now, not after the debt is retired. This is revolutionary information: most of the advice out there is "Pay off your debt as fast as you can, even if it means living on cat food—*dry* cat food."

- *Do whatever you must to pay the bills without borrowing money, but don't discard any viable dreams.* In other words, you might have to take a second job, move to a cheaper place, or sell something you never thought you would, but if you still believe in yourself as an actor or a writer, don't give up on that dream, even if it has to go on a back burner for the time being.

- *Donate 10 percent of all money that comes to you.* Give to the organization that nurtures you spiritually, to a cause that stirs your soul, or to some creative combination. This opens the way for money to flow in from the universe (see chapter 25, "Put 10 Percent to Work for Good").

- *Save 10 percent of all the money that comes to you.* Without savings, you'll never get over the nagging fear of going broke—and unlike a lot of fears, this one would be grounded in reality. If you're terrified, save less for the first few months and work up, but don't dawdle. If you're starting late—i.e., you've already dawdled—bite the bullet and save more (see chapter 26, "Put 10 Percent to Work for You").

- *Have adequate insurance.* The essentials are health insurance (lack of it can lead to financial ruin even if you've done everything else right), property or renter's insurance, and life insurance if you're a parent or if your death would leave your partner in reduced circumstances.

- *Take care of yourself (and minor children if they're in the picture) first.* It's all right to let adult children be adults. It's fine to let the salesman make his commission from the next customer. And since you're already donating 10 percent to the places where you think it should go, you needn't be guilt-tripped into contributing to somebody else's pet cause.

- *Come to see that abundance is allowed,* money isn't evil, and the first step toward doing good in the world is paying your own way.

These basics don't seem boring to me anymore. In fact, they're exciting. They've enabled me to move to New York City, get my daughter launched, not owe anything, and know that, late start and all, things are working out just fine.

Take an Action

Figure your net worth. That's how much you actually have today in savings, stocks, equity in your house or condo, and possessions (such as a car or jewelry) that could easily be turned into cash. Subtract from this what you owe in credit card debt, student loans, money borrowed from other people, and so on. When you have the number, it's simply that: a number. If it's low—even less than zero—understand that it's just providing information, not passing judgment. You're heading up—way up.

Chapter 24

GIVE CASH A CHANCE

You might have credit cards in gold and platinum, but green is still the color of money. The financial experts advise that you pay off your credit cards and get the number in your possession down to one—or even zero if you're undisciplined with credit or if your lifestyle is such that a debit card is fully adequate. However, these learned money folk often couch their one-or-fewer-credit-cards pronouncement with what can seem like a punitive attitude: "You have been bad. You have charged boots and lunches and small appliances. As penance, you must destroy these pleasure-packed cards and take a vow of abstinence from buying anything except groceries." Wow. Let's all do that.

But you know what? There really is a "Wow!" element to living on a cash economy, defined here as spending only money that belongs to you. When you use actual currency, it looks like money. When you spend cash, you are immediately and acutely aware of how much you're trading for the manicure that will last five days, the vitamins that will help you feel healthy for a month, or the tie that your dad won't wear but the thought was nice. A key idea I picked up from *Your Money or Your Life* is that money equals time: if you earn $20 an hour, a $20 expenditure translates into sixty minutes of your time on earth. When you're looking at that bill, fresh and crisp from the ATM, it's easier to see "one hour" than when you're proffering plastic. You become a more discriminating shopper, buying only what you need and what you love. As a result, your wardrobe and your home eventually become more beautiful.

Giving cash a chance—that is, only spending money that is yours *now*—doesn't mean carrying around wads of currency and having more stashed away in sugar bowls and stuffed between the sofa cushions. You can write checks and use a debit card and sign up for automatic bill-pay. It's just that you won't be writing checks for funds that are not in your account, and you'll decline any bailouts from your bank's cash reserve program. Still, in the beginning, using actual government-issued greenbacks whenever possible helps you understand at a visceral level exactly how much it takes to maintain your way of living.

The fundamental gift of a personal cash economy is knowing that what's in your wallet and on the bank receipt, minus outstanding checks, is what you really have. It's easy to stay on top of your finances this way because surprises are minimal and the math is suddenly second-grade simple. You feel strong and responsible and in charge because you're making decisions about where your money goes instead of just shifting bills, chasing checks, and using your Peter card to pay your Paul account.

Cash brings clarity, a trait lacking in the monetary affairs of most people who have difficulty there. They are usually in far worse shape than they're aware of, but every so often you'll hear of someone who's so vague that he doesn't even know he has thousands of dollars in an account somewhere. When you switch to a cash economy, you have to know what you've got: what you're making, what you're spending, and where you stand. This is liberating, even when the numbers start out smaller than you'd like.

When you want something big, you save for it, as archaic as that may sound. Remember how that felt as a kid, buying something with your very own money? It feels just as good now. And it helps you discern, from all the passing fancies out there, what really would upgrade your life.

Getting started on a cash economy is as simple as one-two-three:

1. If you haven't already, find out where you stand right now. Dig out all those icky statements or go online and figure out exactly how much you have and how much you owe. If the results are depressing, take heart: you're on your way to a much healthier plus column.

2. Destroy and cancel all credit cards but one. If you're a chronic debtor, you'll need to get rid of all of them, but for now see how you do with one that you'll pay off in full every month.

3. The following is something I learned from the book I didn't want to read, Jerrold Mundis's *How to Get Out of Debt, Stay Out of Debt, and Live Prosperously*. Write down

every dollar you spend for a month. If you spent more
than you made, you've cut into your net worth. The
idea is to create what Mundis calls a "spending plan"
(less prickly a term than "budget") that covers your
needs and fits within your income. If this is impossible
in your current circumstances, you need to cut expenses
or generate more income by asking for a raise, taking a
second job, getting a gift from someone (not a loan—
that would just get you in deeper), or in some other
clever way bringing more money in.

A realistic spending plan gives you parameters within
which to operate. It shouldn't be tight and unyielding, although even a generous spending plan may seem restrictive if
you're used to buying anything you feel like whenever you
feel like it whether you have the money or not. Give it some
time. Like eating three moderate meals a day, living within
some reasonable financial boundaries will soon feel safer and
more comfortable than profligate spending, with the specter
of broke always waiting in the wings.

Once your spending plan is established, you can operate
on a cash economy—currency, checks, electronic transfers,
debit card. If you choose to keep one credit card activated,
use it judiciously and pay it in full every month. Even better:
pay the bill online weekly or biweekly when you get paid.
(You can also run "to charge or not to charge" for a particular
item past an action partner, just like we did with "to eat or not
to eat" in chapter 19.)

As you continue writing down what you spend, you'll alter
your plan to accommodate the seasons of the year and the

phases of your life when different expenditures are appropriate. This record of where you put your money is a numeric memoir. In seeing where your money goes, you see where your attention goes and what you value. If you like what you see, keep spending precisely as you are. If not, change it. Doing this only *sounds* like renting a room in the chamber of horrors. It's really a great way to assert your independence.

Take an Action

Give cash a chance. If money is problematic in your life, write down every penny that comes in and every penny that goes out for a long enough period that you get a good sense of what's going on in your personal financial dealings. Most people need to do this for a month, a full billing cycle, to get a handle on it. For now, don't worry about spending less; just become aware of what you do spend. Based on this information, create a sensible spending plan for yourself that enables you to live on a cash economy. (For more details, I recommend *How to Get Out of Debt, Stay Out of Debt, and Live Prosperously* by Jerrold Mundis.)

Chapter 25

PUT 10 PERCENT TO WORK FOR GOOD

Many religious people practice tithing, giving 10 percent of whatever money comes to them to their church or some other good cause. Even more intriguing is that many rich people—some of them very, very rich people—have faithfully engaged in tithing and credit the practice for a good deal of their wealth. John D. Rockefeller tithed from early childhood. I once saw a copy of the financial log he kept, "Ledger A," with youthful notations such as, "Received from Father, .10. Given to church, .01." By the end of his life, Rockefeller had given away some $750 million.

Obviously, giving keeps charities and religious institutions going, but it doesn't make sense that giving away 10 percent of your money should help *you* have more. Because it doesn't make sense (and because I really wanted to keep it all), I was an off-and-on tither for years. I'd usually start tithing when money was tight, and having exhausted other options for loosening it up, I figured I'd try giving away 10 percent of the pittances that trickled in. In such a state years ago, I spoke with a minister and told him, "I was paid $200, but after the bills and buying gas and groceries, I have only $20 left. You wouldn't expect me to tithe that, would you?" He said, "In your situation, I think you really have to." I slammed my last twenty bucks down on his desk with the godly phrase "Here's your damn tithe" and stormed out. The next day I received a totally unexpected gift of $500.

Odd coincidences like this one would get me going on tithing, and I'd be a vocal proponent. I'd find the 90 percent going further than 100 percent had gone before. But then something would happen: I'd start bringing in substantially more money than I was used to. I'd get a raise or more freelance work. People who had owed me money for so long I'd given up on it would come through. Every now and then I'd write something that spoke to a reader in a special way and in an envelope from a stranger I'd find a check for $32 or $11.80 and a note saying, "You helped me so I want to send you my tithe."

It was great. Invariably, though, the tithe checks I was writing got too big for my comfort zone. It was one thing to give $20, even when it was all I had. It was quite another to shell out $1,000 or more. I'd be terrified of all those zeroes and give up tithing. Invariably, the zeroes backed off and the money stopped coming.

This happened way too many times for me to write it off as chance. I now believe that tithing is a spiritual law designed to protect human beings and ensure that we'll have all we need. It keeps the flow going. Today it seems to me that that 10 percent off the top needs to get out of my bank account as soon as possible. That first 10 percent is not my money and it's not going to do me any good. If you'd like to experiment with tithing and see what it does for you, here are some common questions and answers as I see them:

Where do you give your tithes? Wherever you're guided. Some experts insist that you tithe to your church or whatever place gives you spiritual nourishment. (Of course, a lot of these experts are providers of spiritual nourishment.) I give more widely than this. Although I do belong to a church and gratefully support it, I also donate to a few select charities and elsewhere as circumstances dictate (if there's a natural disaster somewhere, or a friend is in a charity walkathon).

Do you tithe from the net or the gross? Whatever you're up for. Net makes sense to me since that's what you see. As your consciousness (and your income) expands, you can graduate to gross if you're so inspired. (Some teachers recommend that the self-employed give from their net, after business expenses but before taxes.)

Do I have to tithe from all the money I get or only from what I make at my job? You don't have to tithe at all. If you choose to, it needs to be 10 percent of all income from every source. After all, you want to be receiving income through every channel you can think of and some you don't even know about yet.

What if I get a valuable present that isn't money? Do I tithe on the value? Since we don't use designer watches and laptop computers as currency, simply accept and enjoy the gift. If at any point you sell it, tithe from the proceeds.

Should you tithe if you're in debt? That depends. Ideally, you'll set up a spending plan that includes your tithe *and* a reasonable way to pay back what you owe without living as if you're in debtors' prison. If you're in the midst of a debt crisis (creditors are calling, you're scheduled for court, you've heard wolf-like growling at the door), give only 1 percent of your income right now. Even that will help you feel less desperate: as long as you can give to somebody else, you haven't gone under. Commit to working up to 10 percent as soon as you're out of crisis mode.

What if I miss tithing for a week or a month? Do I have to make it up? If you missed because you were on vacation or otherwise occupied and the earmarked money is there waiting to be donated, by all means stay current. Or maybe you didn't tithe because 10 percent in the hand looked better than a spiritual law in the bush. You spent the money and doing a double-tithe this month would lead to financial hardship. In that case, don't worry about backtracking. Just start again this payday.

I'm married. Should I tithe from what my spouse earns too? Only if he or she understands the process and wants to do it with you. Otherwise, just tithe from what you make. If your spouse is the sole wage-earner and half of his or her income is yours, tithe from your half.

I'm not religious. I feel strange doing a religious thing. Lots of people who aren't religious have discovered the prosperity equation of 10/10/80: give 10 percent, save 10 percent, live well on the remaining eighty. If tithing is too ecclesiastic a term, call it something else, but take advantage of the ease and regularity of 10 percent off the top.

Why does it have to be 10 percent? Why not 8 or 17? Ten has been called "the magical number of increase." It's simple to figure and generations of practitioners attest to its efficacy. If you want to give more than 10 percent and you can do that without defaulting on your responsibilities or sacrificing your needs, give all you like. It may only be zeroes, but those zeroes can do a world of good.

Take an Action

Start tithing with the next money that comes to you—your paycheck, a dividend, the $10 your grandma sends for your birthday. Give with appreciation that you're so rich you can give back.

Chapter 26

PUT 10 PERCENT TO WORK FOR YOU

I hated saving money when I was still little enough for the kiddie rides. Maybe it came from a Cold War childhood and figuring I should live like there's no tomorrow because there might not be one. Or maybe I was just empty inside and believed that buying things would fill me up. Either way, I remember my dad's patient prodding on the issue. He bought me so many banks—pigs and kewpie dolls and globes. The ones with stoppers were great: I could empty them and pocket the cash. Some I had to break to get the money out. Those gave me a moment's hesitation, but ultimately it was always "So long, piggy!"

Once my father got me a super-bank: a miniature airplane of indestructible gunmetal. I'd pull back on the cockpit to deposit each coin, and when I did, the propellers spun in a vain attempt at takeoff. It was okay for a bank, except that it had a key, the whereabouts of which were not revealed to me. I searched and searched. Finally, during a game of race car in the Pontiac (emergency brake engaged, of course), I saw it: attached to the underside of the driver's-side sun visor. I knew Dad would be angry if I took it and he found out, but I figured he had too much important grown-up stuff on his mind to remember the key to a toy bank he'd put there months before. (I was right.) That evening I opened the "baggage compartment" and assessed my loot: $7.80. I felt more guilty than rich, but I spent the money anyway. Even then, broke felt safe in a way that affluent didn't.

This breaking-the-bank pattern continued so far into adulthood that I wouldn't even be telling you this if I didn't believe it would help you. Although I could save for short-range goals—I got a job right out of high school, for instance, and squirreled away enough to move to London—anything long-term was out of the question. Much of my college money went for spas and fat farms (fat, broke & lonely are notorious comminglers). In my twenties, I cashed in a life insurance policy to take a trip or make a purchase—I can't even remember. And a small inheritance that came in my thirties went for I don't know what—student loans, another relocation. Wherever it went, it didn't last long, and I was at home with paycheck-to-paycheck once again.

The only real saving I was able to do was for my daughter's future. Watching her money grow didn't make me nervous; it made me proud. I still couldn't save for myself, but I was getting practice in setting aside part of my income as a matter of course. I figured that when she was taken care of, I could start on me—not an advisable plan, but it was the one I had. By the time it was my turn, I'd learned the formula mentioned in the previous chapter: tithe 10 percent, save 10 percent, live well on 80 percent. I started with those numbers and have worked up to saving a little extra, since I have a twenty-five-year gap to account for.

I might still be spending every penny, however, if I hadn't heard this extremely comforting sentence: "What you save is yours to keep." To most people, this may be as clear as the glass in a Windex commercial, but for me it was groundbreaking. It means that money I save hasn't been stolen from me. It isn't a donation to the bank, and it isn't going into a toy airplane that only my father can open. It is mine to keep—and through the material miracle of compound interest, it will just keep making more with no effort on my part.

Everyone I know who is, if not quite in clover at least in a nice meadow where clover can grow, shares my conviction that saving is the number-one means for keeping broke at bay. Savings are a personal hedge fund: they hedge our bets against future financial difficulties. Having several savings accounts is a good idea. First, there's the tax account, a must if you work for yourself or have freelance income in addition to your regular salary. When you consistently take out money for taxes and Social Security just as if you were the boss (which, if you're self-employed, you are), tax day, whether annual or quarterly, becomes a neutral fifteenth of the month.

Next comes what some people call the "prudent reserve," a savings of around six months' income to get you through an emergency or job loss. Don't panic: it doesn't have to *start* this big. Just plan to build it up. Put these funds in a money market account or even a CD since you won't be drawing on them unless something catastrophic happens.

After the prudent reserve, you'll want to start on (or continue with) retirement savings. If your job has a 401(k) or other retirement plan, sign up. As soon as it's feasible, let those efficient folks in accounting take out the maximum: this is how you can be comfortable (if you're smart about it, outright wealthy) later in life. If you're self-employed, put the max in an SEP or some other IRA. Because history speaks well of the stock market for long-range returns, you'll probably want to put this money in a mutual fund. A financial adviser can help you decide on the particulars. Anything involving stocks still makes me nervous. Maybe I had a prior life and jumped out of a building in 1929. If you relate, having someone in your corner who's knowledgeable about investing is indispensable.

Finally, you can have other accounts for things that are important just to you—a vacation, a sabbatical, a designer something-or-other, whatever you want. I have a savings account for large expenditures related to my business. My husband and I have one fund for a condo (light, spacious, and two full baths, please) and another for the holidays. They've done away with the old-fashioned Christmas club—you'd put in a dollar or two a week and have your shopping money in December—so we've created our own, a savings account to which a regular amount is transferred twice a month. The first time somebody plays "It's Beginning to Look a Lot Like Christmas," we know we're covered for all gifts and apartment staff tips. (Annual tipping is a New York tradition that happens to fall in the most expensive month of the year.) The tree, holiday entertaining, and airfare from Toronto for William's kids are also taken care of. Year-end charitable contributions aren't a burden since we don't make them: year-round tithing takes care of that.

If you're thinking, "This would be great in Fantasyland, but you don't know my situation. I can barely make it through the month, much less put money away. And giving it away besides? Yeah, right." Believe me: I've been there. And to people who started saving and investing when they were twenty, it probably looks like I'm still there. But I'm far from broke, and I feel prosperous. You can too. Start where you are. Get as solid about your financial dealings as the First National Bank and begin to apply the mental prosperity principles I'll outline in the next chapter. Know what you deserve to be making. Even if you have to work for less than that as a temporary thing, envision yourself being paid what you're worth, not years and years from now, but soon enough that you can see it and taste it—just not spend it. We're operating on cash these days, remember.

Take an Action

Quick! Take 10 percent of the money you make and put it somewhere you can't get to it. If some percentage of what you're being paid is already going into a retirement account, start building an emergency fund or prudent reserve on your own.

Chapter 27

EXPECT, AFFIRM, ENVISION

I was waiting for a subway in the Bleecker Street station, reading a book called *Money Magnetism* by J. Donald Walters. I'd read several books with a similar theme: we are created for abundance, poverty is a mistake, and techniques such as tithing and positive thinking can help anyone to a more prosperous life.

Anyhow, I was engrossed in my reading when I felt a tap on my shoulder and realized that a stranger was handing me a dollar bill. I took it to give to the homeless person I presumed it was for, but there was no homeless person. Perplexed, I turned to the benefactor, a young man who pointed at *Money Magnetism*, whispered in my ear, "This stuff really works!" and made his way down the platform. I used the dollar as a bookmark and, after I'd finished reading, passed the book along to a friend and the buck to a street musician.

"This stuff" that "really works" is the notion that we weren't put here to struggle. Nature is a profligate provider. It's part of the right order of things that we have our needs met and acquire whatever is necessary for playing our role on earth at Academy Award level. Way back in the 1920s, Florence Scovel Shinn wrote in *The Game of Life and How to Play It* about a great game of giving and receiving: "Whatever man sends out in word or deed, will return to him.... What man images sooner or later materializes in his affairs.... A person with an imaging faculty trained to image only good, brings into his life 'every righteous desire of his heart'—health, wealth, love, friends, perfect self-expression, his highest ideals."

Too many of us, however, use our imaginations to manifest what we don't want. We think poor. We figure if we haven't made it by forty (or whatever age we pick), we're not going to. We assume that if we didn't come *from* money, we'll never come *to* it in any real and lasting sense. And some otherwise freethinking modernists cling to the old-fashioned concept that having money is somehow wrong—the root of all evil. (Actually, the Bible says that the *love* of money, not money itself, is the problem; that's a big difference.)

To counter the widespread tendency to fear the worst rather than expect the best, metaphysical teachers such as Walters and Shinn offer tools for changing how we think about money in particular and abundance in general. These include:

- *Expectation:* Having the courage to expect the best, even if "best" ends up taking a somewhat different form than you thought it would

- *Affirmation:* Using your auditory sense and your gift of the spoken and written word

- *Visualization:* Employing the sense of sight and your ability to picture what you want, mentally and on paper

Expectation—well-placed expectation, that is—is what you get when you cross faith with positive thinking. It's assuming that things will work out and that what is yours will come to you, even if you run into a detour or setback. People who have a congenitally upbeat nature take to this immediately. The rest of us can recite every horrible thing that's ever happened in history—wars and famines, freak accidents, lovers torn apart—to uphold our vale-of-tears hypothesis.

But just because terrible things *can* happen doesn't mean that wonderful things aren't *supposed* to happen. So you apply for the job expecting to get it. If you don't, know that it wasn't right for you. Call out "Next!" without regret. In another arena, you go on the date assuming that he (she) is either The One or one more karmic dinner accounted for on the way to The One. With positive expectation, the present is as it should be and the future is darned near dazzling.

Affirmation is the making of a positive statement. Formal affirmations are statements that you speak and/or write over and over until you alter a previous thought pattern. Some sample affirmations around money and prosperity are: "Money flows to me easily and freely. I always have more than enough." "My life is peaceful and prosperous. I earn, give, save, and spend wisely and well." "Money is my buddy. We hang out together all the time." "I am a child of God: my dad is rich and so am I." Or make up your own. Just keep it affirmative, present-tense, and certain ("I am solvent and safe" versus "I don't think I'll be broke too much longer").

Affirmations aren't new, and you've probably used them before. If they didn't make a difference for you, it may have been that you were using too many at once, or that you didn't continue the practice long enough. On the three occasions in my life when affirming gave rise to truly spectacular results, I chose one affirmation, wrote it thirty times a day, read it aloud thirty times a day, and kept this routine up for three months. (This is a lot of work. You can see why I've done it only three times.) In addition, I put the affirmation on Post-Its and bookmarks and was so immersed in it that it became true for me even before it happened. (You may be wondering, what were those spectacular results? The first time, I received my biggest book advance to date. The second time, William came into my life. The third time, I was a guest on *The Oprah Winfrey Show.*)

Visualization is seeing the life you want. You can do this as part of your meditation—holding in mind an image of what you want to acquire, achieve, or grow into, or a vision for the world earmarked by peace and well-being.

Another way to use visualization is in the daydreams and imaginings that crop up when your thoughts aren't focused elsewhere. Think for a moment about your free thoughts. (They're like free time, except we haven't gotten too busy to have them.) Where does your mind go when it's allowed to wander? Are you thinking about what you want to build, create, contribute? Are you envisioning a brighter future for yourself, your family, your customers, your community? Or are you more likely to worry? Predict the worst? Mentally rerun the horror flick about the time you were cheated out of money or passed over for a promotion? The movies in your mind are previews of coming attractions—but instead of showing on the small screen inside your head, they'll be full-length features in your life.

A technique for focusing your imaging skills is to craft a vision-map (also known as a treasure-map, mind-map, dream-board, or future-collage). To do this, collect magazines—your own and those of friends and neighbors. (You'll develop a new appreciation for recycling bins in this process.) Leaf through the magazines, cutting out pictures and words that strike a chord with you, that are either literally or symbolically something you would like in your life. Don't edit at this point—assume that you'll probably have more pictures and phrases than you'll use. Keep your clippings in a box or big envelope until you feel you have enough. When you do, arrange the them on a piece of poster board and finalize things with a glue stick. No artistic talent is called for.

Some people like to organize the map by category—financial and material desires in one section, romance and relationships in another, health somewhere else. Other people mix it up. The only "rule" is to put one or more allusions to spirituality, however you interpret that for yourself, in the center of the map. It's a reminder that we're not the focal point of the universe and that life may have its own designs, often far better than ours.

Hang your vision-map where you will see it every day but out of sight of anyone who would mock it. This is a collage of embryonic dreams; they need love and nurture, not teasing or ridicule. Every day look over your map for a full minute or even two. Take it in. I generally make a new map every January and expect to have it up for a year. I kept one four times that long, and every entry on it except one came to pass. I retired the poster when I moved to New York (coming here was one of the visions I'd mapped), and I just might add to my next story-board the one dream that hadn't come true by then—to have a book on the *New York Times* best-seller list.

All those things that happened when I affirmed so intently were also on vision-maps. This kind of double-dipping, although not required, can speed things up. I have found expectation, affirmation, and visualization to be roads to abundance that are, in their own way, just as viable as plugging a debt stream and saving for a rainy (or sunny) day. They operate on a more subtle level, but every good thing starts on a subtle level. Sure, money comes *through* jobs and gifts and grants and interest and all sorts of channels, but it comes *from* the same Source as every other good thing.

Take an Action

Oh, what the heck—take two. First, come up with a prosperity affirmation you like. Write it down and read what you write thirty times (all at once, or ten times every morning, noon, and night) for thirty days. If it doesn't "take" in that amount of time, give it another thirty days, or even ninety like I did. Second, craft a vision-map, hang it up, and make a habit of pondering it for a minute or two every day, inviting into your life both the things you want to have and the person you want to become.

Chapter 28

APPRECIATE NOW, APPRECIATION LATER

I t's a fascinating bit of wordplay that when a stock or a piece of property goes up in value, its worth is said to *appreciate*. When you appreciate what you have at present, your net worth is likely to appreciate as well.

We mentioned gratitude as helpful in breaking up with fat, but it deserves a special place here because there is a straight-line connection between gratitude and abundance. I used to joke that my wallet repelled money. Now I see that the repellent factor was my lack of gratitude for the money and other wonderful things I already had. Like a lot of people, I figured that it wasn't yet time to be grateful, that that would come when I had everything I wanted or was so close to it that being grateful wouldn't jinx my going the rest of the way. I see now that it's *not* being grateful that can jinx you at any stage.

When you were a child, you may have read the children's classic *Hans Brinker, or The Silver Skates*. The book is about a boy in

Holland who wants some snazzy ice skates for Christmas. Instead, his parents give him tulip bulbs. He is, not unexpectedly, disappointed and as irritated as a kid from the olden days is allowed to get. But eventually he figures out that he's supposed to appreciate the bulbs, plant them, and tend them so that they will grow into something beautiful. Once he gets that, he also gets the skates. The message is clear: once you appreciate what you have, more rushes in before you can say triple axel.

Look around you. Where are you right now? In a comfortable home with furniture and appliances and pictures on the walls? In an office that, cubicle though it may be, is evidence that you're gainfully employed? In a café where you just ordered lunch and you'll have money left after you pay for it? You're swimming in a sea of abundance. "But it's not a great big house, and it's not the corner office, and it's not a five-star restaurant." Without the proverbial attitude of gratitude, those wouldn't be enough either. The complaints would just mutate into "But I don't have a second home, and I should own this company, and Maxim's in Paris is so much better than this dump."

You see, ingratitude burrows in and becomes a lifestyle—just like compulsive eating or compulsive spending. Rather than simply acknowledging and envisioning what you want—a positive thing to do—you can get so hooked on what you desire that you're blinded to what you have. I think this is why the Buddhists say that desire is the cause of suffering. The cure for ingratitude (and for a noteworthy amount of suffering, I believe) is found in heavy doses of appreciation.

First, bring to mind all the non-monetary reasons you have to be grateful. Start with your health, the love of the people closest to you, your intelligence, your talents. There's also your ability to laugh and to experience physical pleasure, intellectual delight, and soul qualities like enchantment, wonder, and the certainty you sometimes get that, no matter how things look, you're going to come out smelling like a florist's shop.

Once you're bowled over by all your treasures that money can't buy, move on to the basics it does cover: you have a place to live, clothes to wear, food to eat, and the means for getting from one location to another. Don't gloss over these. *Millions* of people on this planet, and probably quite a few within ten miles of where you sit, don't have a roof or a shower or a guarantee of dinner.

Then start noticing and appreciating the extras—the little quirky things that make you happy. "The tangerine tea I found at the co-op ... my frequent flyer miles ... the tomato plants I put on the fire escape...." Another powerful practice is to express gratitude *for what you don't have yet.* "Thank you for the job I love" is a thought-prayer that, held consistently, could conceivably lead either to a new position or to changes being made where you are so that you end up loving the job you've got.

When you feel grateful, you see how much you have—in fact and in potential. Then you feel rich, and everybody knows the rich get richer. Besides, gratitude is such effective fertilizer that it almost does cause money to grow on trees. This shouldn't be surprising: when given a choice, we go where we're appreciated. Money and the things it can buy do that too.

Gratitude also guards against unnecessary competitiveness and comparing. The tendency to compare yourself to other people can stand between you and an abundant life. When you compare, somebody else always has more or better, although if you could see the other person's situation from the inside out instead of the outside in, it might not look so idyllic. But let's say that it really is idyllic. Let's say the person you're sizing yourself up against truly does have the best of everything in triplicate. Great. This is her life, her role, her destiny. You can't change it (and even wanting to would be like exposing your soul to the flu). You can, however, change your own life by appreciating what you have and being open to the creative ideas that come your way. These ideas are yours to act on for bringing more good into your life.

But what about that other person, the one who seems to have it all already and keeps getting more anyway? What did she do to get where she is? She may not even be that nice. This is a question that has troubled philosophers throughout the ages. The Eastern concept of karma would say that somehow, maybe in a past life, perhaps in some other way, she put forces into motion that created what you see: good looks, loving family, Prada bags, private plane.

Her present obligation is to use what she's been given for the greater good. If she doesn't, her circumstances in a future realm, a future life, or maybe even this one, could be quite different. Your role in this drama is to wish her well. That's also your role in the drama of the homeless person you meet on the street and that of the coworker who is so dead-level even with you that you're sure you have to outdo him to get ahead. No, you don't. You get ahead—in every way that lasts and every way that matters—by striving to be part of the upward progression of the universe. Giving in to the temptation to hold someone back, keep someone down, or steal someone's thunder can only diminish you.

This is where it gets really exciting: the place at which you can be grateful for other people's successes as if they were your own. When you do this, *other people's successes do become your own.* I admit, this is the advanced class, but it is awesome when you can say, "I'm really happy for you," *and mean it.* Once you're there, you get to be happy so much more of the time because you're sharing in the boons of everyone around you. If you've been waiting for a breakthrough to a more prosperous life, here it is. This is where you start to see that riches are far more than bling, ka-ching, and wedding ring. Riches are all around you. When gratitude shows you all you have, it pretty well knocks you sockless.

Take an Action

Don't get out of bed before bringing to mind ten things for which you're grateful. It's just not safe to go out into the world before you've girded yourself with gratitude. There's so much glittery stuff out there to beguile you, not to mention the temptation to believe that someone else has something that's supposed to be yours. Appreciation protects you from these elements the way your winter coat protects you from elements of another sort. How long should you keep doing this exercise? Every morning till you're dead. What comes after that is not my department.

Chapter 29

PUT YOUR MONEY
WHERE YOUR MORALS ARE

The way you use your money is the way you wield your power. Whether you're spending (or donating or investing) $5 or $5 million, you're supporting a way of doing things. Gandhi said, "Be the change you want to see in the world." For good or ill, that could be paraphrased as "Buy the change you want to see in the world." A lot of vested interests are doing just that. But humanity as a whole has an interest in a humane and sustainable world. We need to be pooling our resources in that direction.

Each dollar, pound, euro, yen, yuan, and all the rest is a unit of *energy*. You choose where you want that energy to go. If you think that children laboring in sweatshops is tragic, you'll want to find out where the clothing you buy comes from; otherwise, you could be aiding and abetting the tragedy. If global warming concerns you but you're eyeing a gas-guzzler, you nullify your concern. If war seems to you archaic and absurd but your mutual fund invests in armaments, you're bankrolling the absurdity.

Your purpose on earth is not to take up space and use resources. I detest the phrase "American consumer." It reminds me of flesh-eating bacteria. None of us came here with the life assignment: "Consume all you can." It was instead: "Use your unique gifts and talents to make a positive impact on the world." Your actions are altering the landscape of this planet. You're affecting the future for as long as it will reach. You may be just one person, but history is filled with lone men and women who wrought either enough havoc or enough healing to count for thousands. Be on the healing team—with your thoughts and attitudes, with the direction of your efforts, and with the way you disseminate your capital.

Thoughtful purchasing gives you more power over your money. In addition, spending consciously puts the brakes on spending mindlessly. If you've been writing down where your money goes, as suggested in chapter 24, take a look at those notes. What do you buy and where do you buy it? How much do you know about the companies you routinely support? What kind of world is your money helping create? Do you have any idea who is being helped and who may be suffering as a result of your expenditure? Do you make a point of patronizing businesses whose values echo yours?

In many cases this is a personal call. We all say we want a better world, but we hold different visions of what that would look like. You can be true to yourself and your own ethics only as they stack up at this moment. You can always change your mind or expand your purview as time passes. The following suggestions are a start on using your money to create a kinder, gentler world. Use them to spark your own ideas:

- *Food, glorious food:* Organically grown produce can cost more than the sprayed and petroleum-fertilized variety, but the extra is an investment in a healthier you and a sustainable planet. You support small farmers and save some greenery of your own when you shop at farmers' markets or join a CSA (Community Supported Agriculture) in which you purchase a season's share in an organic family farm. There's information about CSAs at www.localharvest.org.

- *Green, green is green, they say:* Shopping with an eye to the environment is both an enlightening and ennobling experience. Start with packaging, the less the better. Switch to recycled paper towels, and use cloth towels and napkins most of the time. Replace the supplies beneath the kitchen sink with cleansers and detergents that are easier on the environment at large and on your home's environment in particular. (The cheapest way to clean up cleaning up is to use simple products already in your cupboard—baking soda, washing soda, club soda. A book to teach you how is *Clean and Green: The Complete Guide to Nontoxic and Environmentally Sound Housekeeping* by Annie Berthold-Bond.)

- *Energetic expenditures:* Decrease your personal reliance on fossil fuels. Keep your car in tune, get its tires rotated regularly, and don't top off the gas tank. When it's time for a new car, go hybrid. You'll offset the extra cost by what you save on gas. Additionally, there are low-energy furnaces, washing machines, even lightbulbs. Add your actions to those of millions of others, and you'll be part of a positive groundswell.

- *Honor the ma-and-pa:* We depend on large chain retailers, but being able to start and run a business shouldn't be erased from the American Dream. Help keep it alive by seeking out and patronizing ma-and-pa shops, restaurants, and services in your town and when you travel.

- *Secondhand savvy:* I was raised to be a snob about anything secondhand, but not anymore. Vintage clothes are elegant eye-poppers; resale shops can put a girl in Chanel years before her salary would; and plain old used stuff can be totally serviceable, save a bundle, and give new life to something that would otherwise be taking up space in a landfill. Some secondhand stores depress me—the ones that are unkempt and smell musty—but nice ones, such as those run by the Junior League in many cities, are divine. Flea markets, tag sales, eBay, and craigslist are other ways to acquire pre-owned treasures.

- *Inspired investing:* When you put money in the market, research the corporations in which you're considering a partial ownership stake and vow to put your money where your morals are. Sometimes people with an interest in a particular issue buy stock in a company to have input in its direction. Smaller investors can choose from a host of mutual funds under the rubric of *socially conscious* investment vehicles (see www.socialfunds.com for descriptions of the dozens of such funds). Because your social conscience is different from someone else's, you may choose a fund that screens for the "sin stocks" (for example, gambling, alcohol, tobacco), or one that focuses on some combination of environmental awareness, peace, human rights, women's rights, animal rights, and so forth.

- *Charitably choosy:* You can get unbiased information on how your charitable dollars are disbursed from www. guidestar.org, which has financial and operational information on all 1.5 million nonprofits registered with the IRS. If you don't have large sums to give, consider local charities, to which you can donate your time as well as your money. Then you can see how things are being run, and you don't have to trust that the big guys are doing it right.

- *Cease and desist:* Spending makes a statement. Not spending makes a louder one. If you've decided to switch from one product to another because the new one is more environmentally sound, or if you're shopping at a store that has improved its employee relations rather than one that hasn't, let the companies you're boycotting know why they've lost your business and what it will take to get it back.

Have you ever said, "If I had that kind of money, I would ...," followed by some wise, prudent, philanthropic intention? You have the same kind of money as anybody else—the kind that can be used to make things better. When you think of it that way, it feels like a whole lot more.

Take an Action

For the next seven days, diligently monitor where your money goes when it leaves your wallet or your bank account. Notice when your spending seems to you to be promoting a better life for all concerned, when it seems neutral, and when you suspect you're adding to the coffers of a business or industry whose values and objectives clash with yours. Once you see how you're voting with your dollars, take steps to bring your personal integrity to bear on your shopping, sharing, and investing practices.

Chapter 30

CREATE A LIFE THAT INVITES ABUNDANCE

"You should write a book about living rich when you're not," my daughter has told me more than once. "When I was little, I never knew we were poor." I guess I didn't either, even though there was a period when she was six or seven, I was writing articles for low-paying health food–store publications, and little money was finding its way to our little household. We were living at the Lake of the Ozarks in a cedar cabin with one closet between us. (I hadn't realized it was a summer house till winter came and the pipes froze.)

Still, we traveled. I wasn't paid for speaking in those days, but the organizations that sought my services did cover travel expenses for my daughter and me, and I'd add on a day or two so she could see the redwoods or the Smithsonian, the bat colony in Austin or the French Quarter in New Orleans. Back home, we got facials and manicures at the local beauty school for a song. I belonged to the one gym in town, and Rachael (before deciding to go by her middle name, Adair) took tae kwon do there. We belonged to a food co-op, a group of people who ordered organic groceries in bulk, so eating was cheap. Pottery dishes that matched, a glass-front bookcase, the Toyota, and the three cats were holdovers from a more affluent era. The public library, the state park, fascinating friends, and the lake were ours for free. For a while, we even managed to have a cleaning lady.

I take no credit for having lived well on not much. Because I grew up in a fairly well-off family, I saw myself as a person of some means even when I wasn't. Although I'm still doing the work to bring the reality into line with the assumption, I have an advantage in believing that a comfortable life is allowed, even expected. Some people have to overcome different childhood conditioning, the idea of poverty as a family legacy. Someone who grew up amid struggle and lack can make a great deal of money and still see himself as a have-not. A man like this once told me, "No matter how much I make, I always read the right side of the menu first."

If you see yourself as prosperous but you don't have much money right now, you already have the template, like a fill-in-the-dots coloring book you have only to complete. You might admit to a "temporary cash flow problem," but never to being down for the count. If, on the other hand, you see yourself as poor, no amount of stocks and bonds, houses and land, cash and cash equivalents will keep you from feeling poor or fearing poverty. Nothing but your own changed perception will do that. Moreover, this "feeling poor" can go beyond a mere feeling: somebody with a poverty consciousness is hard at work inviting poverty into her life, whether she is aware of it or not. We've all heard of a "reversal of fortune." A downward reversal is more likely for someone who fails to see herself as *fortunate*. Those who do this accept their gifts with gratitude, steward their wealth with wisdom, and share their largesse with love.

Seeing yourself as a person who deserves abundance is the first step toward creating a life that attracts abundance. Thinking and speaking positively, using expectation, affirmation, and visualization, taking a percentage off the top to share and another to save—all these habits help formulate the state of mind that brings good things your way. You have to get chummy with money. Come to know at your very core that your being broke is not going to help one starving child—quite the contrary, in fact.

In addition, you can take some simple, practical steps that will make it easier for abundance to find you. Let's say you're expecting a UPS package. If your house number is easily visible above your front door, or if your name is large and legible by your apartment buzzer, you'll get your parcel today. Otherwise, there might be a time-consuming search for the right place to leave the box. It could even be returned to the sender. The following prosperity measures are signs to the universe that you're supposed to receive abundance, no less than an easy-to-spot address is a sign to the UPS driver that you're supposed to get that delivery.

- *Dress rich.* I don't mean you have be dripping in high-carat rocks and sporting designers' initials all over the place. Just look good: cleaned and pressed, no rips or stains, shoes polished and in good repair. (*Well-heeled* is, after all, a synonym for *wealthy*.)

- *Be flawlessly groomed.* I know an up-and-coming singer who was sent to an exclusive jeweler's to try on the regal diamond necklace she would wear for a benefit performance. "I was so nervous," she confided. "I felt like I didn't belong there. And my nail polish was chipped." As soon as she said this, she figured it out: she didn't have a diva's income yet, but she could have fixed her manicure. So fix your manicure, your hair, your makeup. Check in with the mirror a few times each day to be sure the impression you're giving is first-class all the way.

- *Refrain from desperate acts.* Taking from a hotel a pristine little bottle of shampoo or a freshly wrapped bar of miniature soap is a desperate act. Pocketing packets of Splenda at the coffee place instead of buying a box of them at the supermarket is a desperate act. If it feels like you're getting something for nothing, remember that acting like a beggar never made a big shot.

- *Surround yourself with beauty.* "The rich are different from you and me," one of my mentors paraphrased. "They have more beauty." But it doesn't take money to grow flowers or walk in the woods or on a street with arching trees or historic architecture. The paintings at the art museum are just as breathtaking on Fridays-are-free night as at the $1,000-a-patron premiere. Most cities celebrate summer with Shakespeare in the park, Mozart in the garden, ballet under the stars. You simply have to expend the energy to bring your body to where the beauty is.

- *Make a comfortable home for yourself.* Whether you live in the mansion on the hill or a double-wide behind the Dairy Queen, you will attract abundance by making your home comfortable and inviting. If you're a minimalist, you'll do this by clearing out every iota that's extra and revealing the grace inherent in functionality and open space. If you love collections or antiques or the coziness you feel around throw pillows, crocheted doilies, and stacks and stacks of books, you'll want to weed out the junk from the gems and arrange what's left in a way that nurtures you, body and soul.

- *Live in a great big world.* A great big world is filled with a variety of people, ideas, sights, sounds, and experiences. While money can give you a bigger world with more opportunities to travel, go for advanced degrees, or otherwise enlarge your view of things, it sometimes does the opposite, relegating many of the rich to ghettos of privilege from which they dare not venture out. Be rich in every sense of the word, starting now by living in the biggest world you can create for yourself.

I used to know a fellow named Dennis who taught art part-time at a preschool. The kiln broke in some unfixable way, and the school didn't have the budget for a new one. Dennis replaced it at his own expense. When I complimented him for his generosity, he said, "It's only money, and I'm rich." By most people's standards, he wasn't. He worked as a firefighter and did his art (and art teaching) on the side. He also played in a band, pretty much for drinks and tips, although every time they played a song he'd written it was payday in spades. Dennis owned his home, knew he had a good pension coming from the fire department, and had such wealth in art and music and his own brand of philanthropy that when he said he was rich, he really was. As beauty is in the eye of the beholder, rich is in the mind of the bestower. When you're thinking and living richly, broke has nowhere to hide.

Take an Action

Make a list of ways that you can, with the time, talent, and money at your disposal, redecorate your life so that it invites abundance. These can be elegantly simple. Clearing the clutter from your rooms and closets is an abundance lure. Anything handmade, home-cooked, or fresh from nature puts richness in a space and in a life. So does choosing quality over quantity (and getting to know a shoemaker and a tailor so your quality clothes will last as long as you love them).

Part Four

BREAKING UP WITH LONELY

When your life is full and your spirit engaged,
you'll delight in your own company and draw caring,
supportive people into your world.

Life is all about attraction. You've seen already how you can attract fullness or emptiness, abundance or lack, through what you believe and how you behave. Lethargy, disinterest, negativity, and selfishness decrease your personal magnetism. Alternatively, energy, optimism, and compassion draw creative ideas, inexplicable good fortune, and other energetic, optimistic, compassionate people into your sphere.

Although "lonely" doesn't want you to believe it, you are every bit as entitled to great relationships as you are to wholesome food, a body you enjoy living in, and the wherewithal for a wonderful life. Your most important relationship is with your Higher Power, then with yourself, followed by first-tier others (immediate family and friends so close they may as well be immediate family), second- and third-tier people, and your extended family that consists of all human beings and all living beings. It's wise to cultivate these relationships in order. Often someone will search almost obsessively for a mate, but if they find one and don't yet know themselves, the relationship is handicapped before they get to "What's your middle name?" and "Do you have any brothers or sisters?"

Living without loneliness requires an understanding of personal magnetism. When yours is both strong and discriminating (you want to *attract*, but not everything and everybody), the people who come into your life will be there because they're as terrific as you are. You'll know you're loved, whether you're currently coupled or not. You'll look at "alone" and see "all one."

Chapter 31

LONELY ISN'T FUNNY

We've all been there: lonely because we're alone and lonely when there are people all around but none of them knows us the way we yearn to be known. Because we arrive alone on earth and leave that way too, loneliness is, philosophically speaking, inescapable. But to feel alone because you feel you're somehow lacking just hurts too much.

Lonely comes in layers like an onion that can make you cry. The outer layers are obvious. We live behind closed doors, and we travel in automobiles that may seat five or eight, but we're so often alone in them highway departments decree that one driver and one passenger make a "pool." Someone decided that the nuclear family was sufficient, so we lost the comfort of an extended clan, that village as necessary for raising spirits as for raising a child.

For all the talk of teamwork in the business world, most people's workday is spent behind a desk, behind a screen— and Americans spend more hours a day and more weeks a year there than a European worker would stand for. In the leisure time we've got, most of us aren't gathering like our pioneer ancestors for some updated equivalent of a quilting bee or barn-raising. Instead, we might send an e-mail that says, "R u ok?" and believe we've socialized.

The deeper layers of loneliness respond to the *fact* that we are hopelessly alone until we understand the *truth* that we are inextricably connected. We won't come to this understanding as long as we're looking for connection in a fantasy we concocted long ago. You might crave a Norman Rockwell–style family circle, but Norman himself, married three times and treated for depression, may well have been painting the life he wanted more than the one he had. Or perhaps you're single and convinced that a relationship will give you that sense of being part of something; then you find somebody—and come to see how much space can exist between two people in a double bed. Maybe you felt a beatific companionship with the child you carried and birthed, only to have her reach twelve or thirteen and ask you to pretend you don't know her when you're together at the mall.

There is no question that human relationships are essential for well-being and even physical health. The Harvard Nurses' Health Study (which looked at risk factors for chronic disease in 122,000 women) concluded that the absence of a close confidante is a health risk comparable to smoking. Still, unless we can befriend ourselves, our friends are likely to seem casual rather than close and, despite their best efforts, incapable of taking the loneliness away.

It sounds daunting, and yet the same spiritual connection that can keep you from needing to eat everything in sight or spend your kids' tuition money at Banana Republic can transform loneliness from ordeal to initiation. Spiritually speaking, you are never alone. Admittedly, it takes some doing to transfer that insight from a concept on paper to a conviction in practice, but even playing with the notion that every individual is an expression of a greater whole can help you feel less separate, less subject to the "terminal uniqueness" that keeps us lonely and apart.

At certain times, though, you're just going to feel it. When you move to a new place and don't know a soul. Or when you lose someone close to you, and loneliness and grief double up so you can't tell them apart. Or when your children leave home, a romantic relationship dissolves, or a friendship dissipates. You'll feel loneliness when it seems as though "everybody" is at the shore or the party and you're here, by yourself. Or if you live alone and there's no one around, or you live with people but they're off somewhere (even if the first few hours or days without them brought welcome quiet and privacy). Or when you're with people and feel that you shouldn't be lonely, but those people are so clueless about what's going on inside you, you feel like E.T., desperate to phone home.

The symptoms are painful, but the diagnosis is: you're fine. Anybody would feel lonely under the circumstances. Where it gets troublesome is when lonely uses your preconceptions to keep you under its thumb. You might, for instance, be perfectly content being alone Wednesday, Thursday, or even Friday night, but dreadfully lonely on *Saturday* night because you believe that only losers and ugly people that nobody likes are alone then. It's illogical (you didn't get ugly between Thursday and Saturday), but life is less interested in logic than in molding itself around our beliefs.

It helps to remember that beliefs are subjective. "I'm thirty-eight and not married" can be excruciating to a woman yearning for her soul mate and motherhood, but for one eager to join the Peace Corps, it's a statement of the freedom that will help her dream take shape. When you can keep beliefs and facts discrete, some lonely-provoking situations can be reframed. "My sister is having people over and she didn't invite me" can shift from "She hates me and she doesn't want me to meet her friends" to "Thank goodness—that's one less family obligation."

Loneliness is legitimate. All people feel it. Even dogs feel it; that's why it's a good idea to have more than one. But allowing aloneness (or left-out-ness or guy-less-ness) to erode your self-esteem is not legitimate. When you can't value yourself, you lose yourself, and you're the only friend you really can't do without, even for a little while.

Take an Action

Reach out to someone today. Make a call. Have lunch with another human being. Prince Charming isn't the only person who can assuage loneliness. Give the rest of us a shot at it. And keep up with daily quiet time: your Higher Power never has a previous engagement.

Chapter 32

THE SCORE IS: ENERGY ONE, LONELY NOTHING

Just as misery loves company, lonely loves lethargy, and it tries to suck your energy as if your body/mind/spirit came with a straw. You see, love is an energy, and when you feel it, you aren't tired (well, unless you were up half the night watching a *Special Victims Unit* marathon). If you feel that there isn't love in your life, or that it's not from the right people ("Of course my mother loves me, but your mother has to love you!"), your energy field is missing out on a tremendous source of vitality. Lonely takes advantage of this and tries to convince you that, short of kissing the right frog, you'll never feel motivated or impassioned again. You may as well take a nap. Till next week.

Friendship, which is just love in pastels, is another source of energy. The human body is an electrical machine, an energetic organism. When you're in contact with another person—not necessarily in an intimate sense, just sitting across a table and sharing conversation and a blueberry scone—you partake of that other person's energy. The exchange nets a mutual gain. When you aren't making this kind of human contact, you have to draw on your reserves. Natural introverts can self-energize in a way that extroverts can't, but everybody requires some amount of "other" energy. When it's lacking and your reserves are low—in other words, when you're lonely—you have to offset the energy shortfall.

One response is to ingest exogenous energy—coffee didn't get to be a sacred herb for nothing—but ultimately the energy has to come from inside you. If you're feeling lonely, lethargic, and generally pitiful about the state of your life, pull yourself up by your sandal straps and either get out or stay in and do something creative or something rewarding. I promise this will generate energy. When it does, you may forget that you were lonely in the first place, either because you've connected with people or because you're feeling so good about yourself that you don't need anybody else around right now.

There's a continuum here. It's not a matter of *either* "lie on the couch and feel dejected" *or* "move your butt and experience ecstasy." You are a complex, cyclic, multifaceted being. Sometimes you want to shut out the world and chill all weekend; other times twenty minutes by yourself feels like banishment. During a bona fide down period, neither shopping the sales nor volunteering at a soup kitchen is likely to reconfigure the brain chemicals, planetary influences, time of the month, or whatever the hell it is that makes getting through this day feel like wading through sludge. It does, however, inject movement into the scenario, and sometimes a little movement is enough to start to turn things around.

"A little movement" could mean scrolling up through the big channels to find an inspiring movie instead of watching old episodes of *Hollywood Squares* because you're too listless to operate the remote. It could be going to the kitchen and making yourself a cup of tea instead of lying around thinking how nice it would be if someone made you a cup of tea. A little movement might be making a phone call, or reading a magazine, or planning what you'll do when you're up for doing something. Just thinking about what you'd really like to be doing stirs some of that dormant energy.

When you have even a tiny bit of vitality to work with, invest it in a way that generates more. Physical movement—exercise—is a great place to start. It creates endorphins, the safe and legal uppers the body prescribes for itself. Exercise also boosts your self-concept. If you can drag yourself to the gym and into the Cardio Latino class, coming home to a houseplant (or a person who's as communicative as a house-plant) won't seem so lonely.

Another surefire energy enhancer is to shower yourself with self-care. The luxurious aspects of self-care are usually the first casualty of a lonely invasion, with basic maintenance not far behind. In the best of possible worlds, you could meet loneliness head-on every time with one of those "days of beauty" at a spa. Seven and a half hours of washing, cutting, coloring, massaging, steaming, waxing, filing, massaging, pol-ishing, pampering, primping, massaging—who needs a boy-friend when life is this good?

All right, so your great-grandfather didn't found a chain of hotels, and most of the time you'll have to deal with loneliness in a less extravagant fashion. Still, the example underscores the contention: taking care of your body does wonders for your psyche. Remember: loneliness is just a fact of being, like getting thirsty or having your foot fall asleep, until you compound it with shame and self-abandonment. A facial mask, professional or self-administered, tells lonely that you know you count. Then it backs off.

Organizing and fixing up your place is another way to assert that although you may be by yourself, lonely doesn't need to drop in for a visit. Eating really delicious, really healthful food is also a key tactic. If you're feeling lonely or downhearted, scaling tall buildings in a single bound can seem easier than washing lettuce. Do what you need to: buy salad in a bag, all washed and ready. Go out to eat. If you have to nuke something, at least serve it on a plate. I don't know why this is, but lonely loves having dinner on paper, plastic, or Styrofoam.

Poetry and the spiritual writings from around the world can feed your soul and build your momentum. Music (the kind you absolutely love, not the CDs your former fiancé hasn't come by to claim yet) is another ally. Some people go for lyrics, others for orchestration. To be therapeutic, music has to reflect your preference. I mean, Mozart is sweet like soy chai in the morning, but to nudge me out of a lonely spot I need the cheesy but moving instructions I get from musical theater when it tells me to "climb every mountain," "dream the impossible dream" and, "when you walk through a storm, hold your head up high." Of course, if you can make your own music—piano, guitar, Flutophone—do it. The song could be a hundred years old, but when you play it, it's a rendition being heard for the very first time. That's energizing. Singing is good too, and the great thing about singing when you're alone is that nobody comments if you sideswipe a note.

Finally, there's God (or any of the synonyms from chapter 8)—not as some faraway, up-in-the-sky deity, but a Presence that's inside you all the time. I know God won't rub your back or tell you how amazing you look, but if God is indeed Love, He/She/It ought to be pretty darned adept at making you feel loved. Let Him (Her/It) do that. When you feel loved deep within yourself, you attract love from other people. Open yourself up to the idea that your Higher Power is hopelessly in love with you and has been for, jeez, all your life? Since the beginning of time? And that love has never once faltered, no matter how much you ate or who you slept with or how bitchy or whiny or selfish you ever got. This is one major love. It is, in fact, *the* major love. When you allow yourself to feel it, your whole life changes. And you'll radiate a kind of caring that draws other people to you.

Techniques like these aren't just self-help-in-a-jar. They stoke energy the way a well-positioned bellows stokes a fire. The lazy, can't-get-out-and-don't-really-care response puts you just where lonely wants you. If instead you recoup your energy daily and build your reserve supply, lonely can't get you because it can't catch you. One caveat: if you're experiencing a lack of energy and enthusiasm for life that's gone beyond a temporary lonely spell, there could be a treatable, biochemical reason why getting out of your bathrobe doesn't seem worth the effort. If this is the case, getting professional help is the smartest, kindest thing you can do for yourself. Whatever you need to do, don't take this lying down—and I mean that literally.

Take an Action

As long as you keep your energy up, lonely can't keep you down. Without energy, you can fall into isolation: "I'm lonely.... Gosh, I feel tired. I guess I'll stay in.... Oh shoot, who's calling me? The voice mail can pick it up." After a few go-rounds, the phone stops ringing, and even when you want to do something fun or productive, it can be hard to think of something fun or productive to do. Therefore, your action to take is to make a list (when you're not in a funk) of everything that makes you feel empowered and alive. Put copies of your energizing list in every possible place—fridge, medicine chest, desk drawer, nightstand, "My Documents"—because when you're feeling lonely and despondent, you may not even remember you made the list if you don't happen on it inadvertently.

Chapter 33

FALL IN LOVE WITH YOUR OWN COMPANY

Oscar Wilde advised falling in love with yourself as "the beginning of a lifelong romance." This thought doesn't sit well with certain people. To some it implies conceit, to others a concession to never being loved by some marvelous other person. In fact, it's nothing of the sort. To deal with life's inevitable loneliness with as much grace as possible and as little pain as necessary, you have to fall in love, if not with the sound of your voice and the size of your thighs, certainly with your own companionship. This is nothing but being a good friend—to yourself.

What makes a good friend? Well, being kind and funny and dependable and being someone who likes to do the things you both enjoy. Since the two of you—or, in this case, the one of you—already like the same stuff, all you have to be is kind and funny and dependable.

Kindness is just love with its work boots on. You extend it to yourself by treating yourself as well as you treat other people. If you smile at strangers on the street, smile at yourself in the mirror. If you'd serve a guest something better than peanut butter out of the jar, do the same for yourself. If you'd tell a child that spilling milk is no big deal, tell yourself that when you spill wine. Even red.

As for *funny*, just have fun. The ha-ha stuff will make its way in. Teenage girls aren't masters of wit and comic timing, but they can giggle for an extended period because they're willing to get silly and the culture allows it. Be willing to have fun and be funny, and don't give a whit about who allows it and who doesn't. A very funny person I know, comedian Wendy Spero, author of *Microthrills: True Stories from a Life of Small Highs*, once had an executive assistant job in a straitlaced corporation. To put some literal sparkle into the day, she would routinely add glitter to her boss's reports and memos. He came to look forward to the diversion of sparkling specks in the midst of boilerplate boredom. His superiors didn't get it. Their loss.

I used to think that laughter and fun were extras, like dessert. Now I believe they provide essential nutrients. You owe it to yourself to have some fun every day. No one knows what the future holds. The fun you have today goes into a memory vault where you can pull it out when you're under a rain cloud like Eeyore in *Winnie the Pooh*. If you keep a journal, I suggest that you write down every night at bedtime something fun that you did that day. It doesn't have to be uproarious. "Saw a movie" works. So does "Drank bubble-tea" or "Did the crossword with my kid."

Quite a few people, myself among them, are not innately gifted in the fun department. Playing makes us nervous. I recently saw how recreationally challenged I am when I took an improvisational comedy class through Chicago's legendary Second City. It involved three hours of agonizing "games" every day for a week. I so wanted to quit, but I stuck it out. (When you write self-help books, you do have to maintain certain minimal standards.)

In the class, we had to pretend to play catch with an invisible ball ("You know it's coming to you through eye contact!") and then heighten the stakes with an invisible dagger, being tossed simultaneously. All the throwing and catching and eye contact made my head spin—*because I was taking it all so seriously.* In fact, I was not going to be stabbed. I wouldn't even have to chase an errant ball because there was no ball. That's when it clicked for me: play means letting go of what's real (or what seems to be real) and living in another reality where even winning and losing are make-believe. When you can carry that playful attitude into regular days, the rejections and disappointments that crop up are easier to respond to and bounce back from. And being alone is perfectly pleasant because you're in such delightful company.

Dependability is showing up for yourself. Being in your own corner. You'd think we'd do this as a matter of course, but in the same way that we sometimes fail to be there for others—it's inconvenient or we're tired or overscheduled—we go AWOL in our most basic relationship, the one with ourselves. Reporting for duty in this case involves taking care of yourself, sleeping enough, keeping your clutter down, and making time for things you like to do even when it requires editing something else out of your PDA. It's living each day in such a way that you can look back each night and say, "I did a decent job of it."

Dependability boils down to keeping the promises you make to yourself and not making promises you aren't prepared to keep. "I can only show up for myself in the sphere of what I can control," says Susan Cheever, author of *American Bloomsbury.* "A lot of showing up is in small but esteemable acts: being on time, paying the bills, saying 'I'm not eating sugar today' and then not eating sugar." This kind of behavior results in self-approval and self-respect.

When you become kind, funny, and dependable with yourself, you're more likely to see solitary hours as time well spent. Then you're ready to experiment with planning an evening at home in your own company. You'll do this not because you don't have a better offer but because you've blocked out hours on your calendar to be with yourself and enjoy yourself in some splendidly singular fashion. Maybe you'll rent a film with subtitles, or reread *Wuthering Heights* cover to cover, or deep-condition your hair and give yourself a facial.

After a successful planned evening of "home alone," graduate to the date-for-one. You can go out to dinner and to a movie or a play (single tickets often end up being the best seats in the house). The idea is to have a good time and get over the notion that there is any stigma around not having a date or an entourage.

In case you're worried about ill effects that could arise from self-appreciation, let me assure you that falling in love with your own company will not relegate you to a life of unattached isolation. The opposite is true. You'll be honing your skills for kindness, humor, and dependability, making every relationship in your life, romantic and platonic, richer. These aptitudes and the aura of confidence you'll emanate will draw people to you—and they won't be the needy types who are attracted to others' Sturm und Drang the way sharks are attracted to the wounded. You can expect really terrific people to start to fall in love with your company. You just have to be the first to do it.

Take an Action

Plan an evening home alone that is so deliciously indulgent that you can hardly wait for it to begin. Alternatively (or, ideally, in addition), go out on a date-for-one. Dress nicely but not provocatively and stay out of pickup joints. You already have a date, and you may just be falling in love.

Chapter 34

SEX AND THE GRITTY

Spiritually, you've been commissioned to learn how to love and extend that love in every way possible. It can get complicated when we're talking about the other kind of love, the hearts-and-flowers, my-God-he's-incredible, I-almost-ripped-his-clothes-off-in-the-restaurant variety. If you extend *that* love in every way possible, you really won't respect yourself in the morning—or feel any less empty inside.

When passionate, partnered love is not a present reality in your life, the loneliness can be emotionally devastating and physically painful. It's probably most acute right after a breakup, when there's all of a sudden emptiness in the space where there was so recently a warm, sexy body. (He may not have seemed outrageously attractive when he was here, but let him leave—or find another woman, heaven forbid—and you're sure *People* magazine is going to name him "Sexiest Man Alive.") You can also feel lonely when you've been single for a while and are finding it hard not to project to forever. It can even show up if you're in a relationship that's not meeting all your needs and you think you'd feel less lonely on your own.

After my first husband died when I was thirty-seven, I dated way too soon and way too desperately. I wanted to re-store the "husband piece," to re-create a fully populated family unit. I wanted it with such impatience and intensity that it interfered with my own grieving process. It meant that I was, to my lasting regret, not as available to my little girl as I should have been when she needed me most. And I scared away the men I did meet because they weren't looking to be replacement parts.

I dated one fellow for a couple of years. Sufficiently smitten, I set a goal to get him to the altar. As if I were going for a mas-ter's degree or trying to double my income by a certain date, I was determined to marry this man. He had other ideas and ulti-mately left me for someone he said was "lower maintenance." I felt like a condominium, traded in for one with cheaper carry-ing charges. The loss, so closely following an even greater loss, was intense, and the loneliness almost unbearable.

In retrospective brilliance (we all get so wise after the fact), I see that I should have confronted the loneliness in the ways we've discussed: understanding that it's not fun but that it can be a teacher, keeping my energy up so that I could be lonely but not bereft, and learning to appreciate everyone who was in my life and fall in love with my own company. Instead, I found another boyfriend. When it didn't work out with him either, I said yes to the next guy who showed up and moved with my daughter and the three cats from Missouri to Connecticut.

He was a terrific person, and at the time I believed with all my heart that I was looking for a better life for all concerned.

What I was really looking for, however, was a way to escape: to escape grieving the loss of my husband and to escape the reality that I was a single mom who needed to grow into emotional and financial independence. Of course sex played into it, and sex—as wonderful and magical as it certainly is—can also be as addictive as cookies and credit cards.

Several years ago, an American Sikh told me that her teacher, the late Yogi Bhajan, believed that a woman holds any lover, a one-night-stand included, in her aura for seven years. I wasn't sure I believed in auras, but the thought of some of the guys who might be in there gave me the creeps. That image made it easier, at least some of the time, to fall asleep hugging a teddy bear and to respond to biological urges with a vibrator.

Astoundingly, this kind of independence can get you more attention than high heels, spray-on pheromones, and new boobs from the best surgeon in town. Determined self-sufficiency is a potent aphrodisiac and more than that: it makes your whole *life* attractive, bringing potential *life* partners, rather than simply sexual partners, into your circle.

If I were to give one piece of practical advice to a single person, male or female, it would be to slice off a chunk of the American Dream and buy a house. If you're not prepared to do this or you're not interested in buying a house, or if you already have one, you can translate this suggestion into something else that suggests independence and self-sufficiency for you. Maybe it's starting a business, taking a big trip on your own, or doing some rigorous and challenging volunteer work. Whatever you do, however, has to be as momentous and as obvious as if it had a garage and a basement.

When I was a mere maiden of nineteen, I worked with a woman who was thirty-two and single. She thought that since she'd probably missed the marriage boat (it used to sail quite a bit earlier than it does now), she would buy a house so she'd have financial security. Wham! The ink had hardly dried on the mortgage papers before a fellow who'd done business with our office for years asked her out for the first time. Before she turned thirty-three, they were wed. He sold his house and moved into hers.

Years later I had a similar experience myself. I'd been single for almost a decade. (The Connecticut relationship had gone on longer than most, but it eventually went belly-up like all the others.) One Thursday afternoon I sat down with a cup of Earl Grey and took stock. Although I'd been visualizing and affirming for more of what I wanted, I realized that my life was quite agreeable just as it was. My thirteen-year-old daughter was the light of my life: bright and gifted, with principles she stood for. I was blessed beyond belief in getting to write for a living. And I owned a home. It wasn't my dream house, but it was my house, and on that particular Thursday afternoon it was sufficient. I didn't need anything else, even Mr. Wonderful. I was content, probably for the first time in nine years.

Four days later, I met William.

The skeptics can claim coincidence, but I am certain that without becoming content with my life as it was, it wouldn't have happened. It's that law of attraction in yet another guise: when you feel complete, you attract other complete people. When you don't, you attract others looking to fill their own emptiness, or you attract no one at all.

The same principles apply when you are in a relationship. That old phrase "my other half" is quaint, but nobody wants to be married to half a person, and being half a person is even worse. You have to know who you are and love you who are. (That's why you just waded through three chapters in this section that don't have to do with another person or other people.) Even though your relationship with your partner should meet enough of your needs that you want to do the work (and there's plenty of it) to sustain that relationship, you're asking for trouble if you expect one human being to play the be-all-and-end-all role.

Obviously, you'll want to get your sexual needs met with this person. That means asking for what you want, making compromises, and trying things that would get you a semester of detention back at St. Cecilia's. You need to have enough interests in common with your partner that you don't fall into the stereotypical "old married couple" picture of the silent dinner suggestive of parallel lives that long since ceased enlivening each other. Open communication is mandatory, and if you don't have it, you need to take a class or see a counselor who can teach you the skills of kind, clear communicating. It's essential not just to hear words but to hear what this person who loves you is actually attempting to say. (This is true for both partners, of course.)

It is imperative that you and your mate have a compatible worldview and are willing to give the other person's dreams the same priority you give your own. But if your honey doesn't like skiing or snorkeling or sushi, you need to be able to pursue these interests on your own or have other people in your life to do them with you—preferably not a straight guy to whom you're incredibly attracted. (Gay women and men of whatever persuasion, please translate to fit.)

As far as I can tell about partnering, it's amazing that it ever happens at all. Nevertheless, you hear stories about people from far-flung countries meeting one another, and about high school sweethearts reuniting in their retirement years. It's no wonder the notion of romance persists and we get all gushy about it. But it's not a matter of glass slippers and blue-blooded frogs: it's about coming into your own so thoroughly that you can meet someone who's done the same.

There are no guarantees. But finding your center, being your own person, and owning your own life (maybe even your own real estate) are ways to increase the odds of meeting someone who's right for you and having a joy-filled relationship once you do. Finding your center, being your own person, and owning your own life also provide great joy and satisfaction whether you're in a relationship or not. A reader of my earlier books, Sharmaine Hobbs, e-mailed me the following when she heard I was writing *Fat, Broke & Lonely No More:* "It used to ache to the bone because I wanted to share my life with a partner so much. I've embraced my singleness, and filled it with life purpose and gratitude for what is rather than what is not."

If you are married or otherwise hitched, the same principles apply. Create a vibrant and viable life for yourself. You'll have more to bring to the relationship and something that's yours should the relationship end. It's as close to happily ever after as you're going to get without a fairy godmother and a four-door pumpkin.

Take an Action

Whether you're in a relationship, looking for one, or on your own for now and content with that, do something today that makes you feel whole. You could put in a garden. Or sponsor a little girl or boy through Save the Children or a similar organization. You could buy a pink flowered sofa because you're single and you can. Or go to an open house and try on the notion that you could own the place. Whatever you opt to do is right, as long as it plants you more firmly in your own good life.

Chapter 35

HISTORY WITH DRUNKS AND LOSERS? DON'T LET HISTORY REPEAT ITSELF

When a friend is in a risky relationship, the rest of us rival Solomon in our sagacity. "There she goes again.... What does she see in him?... That guy has 'bad news' written all over his face...." Yes, we are the voice of reason until we ourselves fall for somebody dangerous. If you haven't done it, you're either darned lucky or you did something really remarkable in a previous life and karma is giving you a free pass. Drunks, losers, and bad boys, the unavailable and the commitment-phobic, guys (and women) who are narcissistic, jealous, brooding, controlling—all the qualities you'd never say you were looking for when you put your profile on MySpace—can be as enticing as your mom's Christmas fudge or a gold card with a 0 percent introductory offer.

We grew up swooning over romantic leads who were almost always a little dangerous. Ashley was a simpering wimp compared to Rhett, and Arthur a geriatric bore in the chivalrous shadow of Lancelot. We love these stories because we love excitement and adrenaline and getting near the edge. I mean, when was the last time you heard of an amusement park advertising its smaller, slower roller-coasters? Now, I am not down on excitement in the slightest. I've gone bungee-jumping, for heaven's sake. But bungee-jumping—and sky-diving, adventure vacations, and extreme sports—are rocking-chair safe compared to giving your heart to someone who doesn't have the personal credentials to handle it with sufficient care.

A great catch is not somebody whose primary appeal is that when he's nice, he's very, very nice. Those little highly charged hints from his dark side that you see early on foreshadow lots more of the same underneath. This doesn't mean you're dating a psychopath. It's just that everybody is on good behavior in the first few weeks or months of a relationship. What you see a little of early, you'll see a lot of later.

Pay particular attention if you've been in several unfortunate relationships of the same type. It could be said, "Into each life, one lush must fall," but two or three or four means you've put out a psychic sign that says, "DRUNKS WELCOME HERE." Ditto for any guy who is in the least bit abusive, or who takes you for granted, or who tells you his wife doesn't understand him and he'll leave her the first minute he's able. He was *able* before he met you. Get out before you grow accustomed to being a chump.

Once you take on that moniker, you're likely to fall prey to serial suckiness. This means that you may not even get the educational value of *different kinds* of dysfunctional relationships. It's just the same one over and over with only the names and costumes changed. Even if you've never dated someone weird enough to get you on a TV talk show, this scenario is still discouraging and disheartening and a huge time-waster. Should you relate, practice speed-dating by speedily exiting the not-right relationship, taking a little time off to process what you learned, and reentering the world of romance stronger and smarter next time around.

Not repeating a history with drunks and losers (or whatever history you'd rather not reenact) is a metaphor for everything you're doing to give fat, broke & lonely its walking papers. If you ate in a way that caused you discomfort and remorse, you can make different food choices. If you used money in a way that made you unsafe and insecure, you can take a different course. And if you were attracted to people who made your heart skip beats but left you feeling sick to your stomach, you can pick different people.

Understand: if you've been attracted to a particular "type" of wrong guy or girl, that type will still turn your head. There is now information *in* your head, however, that this is not fate, love at first sight, or the preordained meeting with your true soul mate who has tragically been drawn into Internet porn and compulsive gambling. Being filed in your brain-computer at this minute are relevant facts: (a) you are *not* gifted with supernatural powers that can exorcise his devils; (b) the promised land is *not* the third-floor walkup you'll share with him after you put down the first month's rent and security deposit; and (c) you will *not* make it all work with the two girls and a boy you'll have together after his vasectomy gets reversed. Of course you'll feel fluttery about this latter-day James Dean. Just feel it—fluttery is an undeniably pleasant sensation—and let it go at that. Imagine tattooed onto your frontal lobe: "Adrenaline is not a sex hormone. It is possible to have deliciously indecent sex with a very decent person."

It's probably easier to work in a chocolate factory and never lick your fingers than to let go of a warm body that's willing to be there for you, even some of the time. But settling extracts a higher price. Getting involved with a practicing alcoholic or drug user, a person with a history of violence, or someone who's been genuinely cruel to you or anybody else, even verbally, is betting on a lame horse. You're not going to win. You also don't want to stay stuck in a ghost town of a relationship, where all your hopes for a future have disappeared but hanging around seems easier than moving on. Getting involved with someone you plan on changing in one or more major ways is pointless too, because you can't change anybody except yourself and even that is not for sissies.

Finally, going forward with any relationship against your dependable intuition is asking for trouble. When you're in the first blush of lust and your friends are telling you how lucky you are, it's almost impossible to even sense a misgiving. If you do sense one, though, even a tiny one, be very aware of it. It could be nothing more than a case of nerves about something new, something fantastic that you think you might not deserve, or it could be a warning you'll be glad you heeded. If you're not sure, don't bolt. Just be alert. And discuss your apprehensions with someone you trust. That way, should love make you blind, there'll be someone around with 20/20 vision.

It is vital, however, to see the difference between settling for someone you would do well to steer clear of and coming face-to-face with a fabulous, albeit imperfect, person who might make a terrific partner in this imperfect world. If there is such a thing as soul mates, yours will (or did) come from the ranks of the fabulous but imperfect. Such a person will love you the best he can and wish he could do it better. This is someone who'll share some of your interests and have some of his own that may be incomprehensible. He might be someone whose mother didn't tell him to turn out the lights when he left a room, even though yours pounded that message home like a one-woman EPA. He's a human being who can't read your mind and who doesn't know until you tell him that saying, "What you should really do ...," makes you want to scratch his eyes out. This fabulous, imperfect person, like all the fabulous, imperfect people you'll meet along the way, has had a life of his or her own up to now. Your entering won't erase what's gone before, and if you take this person into your life, the backstory comes too.

Even a knight in shining armor probably has some post-traumatic stress disorder from all the battles and a little premature arthritis from spending too much time on a horse. That's the way it is with us mortals. Life bats us about, and we find one another at varying stages of injury and repair. You can have a wonderful life with someone who isn't perfect, but he does need to be pretty terrific and remember every day that you're the best thing that ever happened to him.

Take an Action

Go over your relationship history. Are you seeing a lot of "drunks and losers" there, or some other assemblage of folks with limitations you'd rather not have to deal with again? Make a list of the qualities you would like to see in the people you're around—in a romantic partner if you're in the market for one, but also in your friends and even in the coworkers, neighbors, professionals, and service providers with whom you interact. When you know what you're looking for, you will become more discerning. You'll gravitate toward people who have the characteristics you've cited, and more of them will find their way to you.

Chapter 36

YOU'D BE SO NICE
TO COME HOME TO

"**U**mm," the $10 palm reader in Central Park grunted as he simultaneously plumbed my psyche and fed a squirrel. "Is no easy to be man marry to you." I felt like paying him only $7.50, but I needed the reminder that I can be self-absorbed, grandiose, and inflexible—in other words, not always a treat to come home to. But to get lonely a ticket out of town—and to make the most of a relationship when you're in one—you and I and anybody else who's interested has to learn to be relatively easy to get along with.

This would be obvious had we not been overtaught the virtues of looking out for number one. We've read the books and articles that warn against being a pushover. We know that nice girls don't win or hold court in corner offices, and only in the sappy movies do they ever get the guy. We've earned our black belt in vocal self-defense: "This is totally unacceptable." "What part of 'no' do you not understand?" "I have made my decision, and my decision is final."

Assertiveness skills come in handy. No living person, male or female, has been genetically modified with doormat genes, and everyone deserves to be respected and treated well. "Respected and treated well," however, does not translate as being the center of the universe and always getting your way. Camaraderie calls for seeing beyond your nose—and even beyond your needs if you have eleven-hundred of them and not one is negotiable.

To become the sort of person who's nice to come home to (or share an office with, or have on the next mat at Pilates), you only have to learn and practice some simple techniques:

- *Try seeing the world from the other person's point of view.* There's an Indian story about blind men describing an elephant. The one who touches the trunk says, "An elephant is like a snake." The man who touches the tail is sure that an elephant is like a broom. The third, touching the animal's side, is convinced that an elephant is like a wall. Similarly, we all see situations from our personal vantage point. In many differences of opinion, it's not about right or wrong but about where we touched the elephant.

- *Let grievances age for a day.* If you have a catalog of complaints to reel off in the interest of "sharing," let them age for a day. Should you still need to discuss them, by all means do, but if twenty-four hours' distance makes them seem more petty than pressing, let them go.

- *Do sweet little things because they mean a lot.* Everyone appreciates a reminder that they're being thought of. Making the coffee, clipping an article or cartoon, or putting a note in his suitcase when your beau goes out of town isn't a grand gesture, but it means a lot just the same. Try to come up with a little thing that seems as sweet to the other person as to you. For example, I like it when William brings me fresh juice from the deli; he wants me to bring him Diet Coke.

- *Be sensitive to the other person's state of mind.* When your mate (or anyone else, for that matter) is going through a hard time, joining in and making it a blues duet won't help, but your becoming a Comedy Central solo act probably won't either. *Sense* what's needed from you. Would talking help, or listening? Is having you nearby a quiet comfort, or would he or she rather be alone for a while?

- *Make light.* There's so much serious stuff all over: it's on CNN and in business-sized envelopes, in the doctor's examining room and the boss's office. Some of it gets into relationships too—paying the bills, cleaning the house—but the more lightness and fun you can inject into your time together, the more precious you'll become to one another.

- *Don't compete.* If you enjoy competition, take up tennis or golf or poker. In relationships, however, competition is Russian roulette. Forget about who's earning more, who's in better shape, and which one of you the cat

likes better. In any competition, somebody loses and
losing hurts. Besides, you have a spiritual life now.
You're learning that there's enough for everybody.
Success isn't rationed by street address. You and your
fella can both shine. So can you and your sister, and
you and your best friend.

- *Know your stretching limit: go that far and then stop.* Let's say
  you don't like baseball but your true love is a major
  Cardinals fan. How many games can you go to each
  year and enjoy them? How many nights of an extended
  summer are you willing to spend watching baseball on
  TV? Do that much. Wear the hat and the T-shirt and
  be a sport about the sport *until just before you start to feel put
  upon.* When you reach your stretching limit—maybe
  thirty games, maybe three—buy your honey some
  peanuts and Crackerjack and go do something that fills
  you up.

- *Take care of yourself so somebody else won't have to.* When you
  make sure that meditation and exercise don't slide,
  when you eat well and get enough sleep, your well-
  being will be reflected in your mood. In addition, find
  ways to express your talents and engage in the activities
  that make you come alive. This liveliness will infuse all
  your interpersonal interactions and free the people
  close to you to go for the best they know of too.

- *Learn the difference between "big" and "little."* Babies learn these
  words right after *dada, mama,* and *bye-bye,* but grown-ups
  in relationships often can't tell them apart. Robbing a

bank is big; not stopping to buy paper towels is little. Causing you bodily harm is big; eating the last yogurt in the fridge is little. Although there are very few big things, there is apparently no end to the minor irritations people can cause one another. If you fought over all of them, there would no time for sex, or shopping, or planning your next vacation.

- *If you're going to fight, fight fair.* Yelling and name-calling and threats aren't fair. Neither is clamming up and reenacting a good old-fashioned Amish shunning. Bringing up the past or the other person's emotional pressure-points is hitting below the belt. You're supposed to be having a discussion, not going for the featherweight title. Even when you are at odds, remember that you're talking to someone you care about. Besides, if you avoid sarcasm and verbal jabs, you won't have to apologize for them later.

- *Hold your partner and your friends in the Light.* If you're a praying person, pray for the people in your life. Otherwise, send them good thoughts. Visualize them enjoying positive outcomes and realizing dreams.

I am aware, as you are, that these suggestions are not hot new findings from some hot new study. They're commonsense ways of relating that have become a lot less common than they ought to be. They can cover for a multitude of short-comings, even those that might be etched in the palm of your hand.

Take an Action

For the next forty-eight hours, be exceedingly easy to get along with—in your primary relationship if you're in one, and with everybody else besides. This means not having to be right, or have the last word, or get exactly what you want. For two days, you're going to listen more than talk and work harder at understanding than at getting your point across.

Chapter 37

HOW TO WIN FRIENDS AND PUT UP WITH PEOPLE

If the pressure to be in an idyllic relationship isn't severe enough, there's always the pressure to have dozens of idyllic friendships. From Lucy and Ethel to Laverne and Shirley to Will and Grace, we've been told that having a bestest-bestest friend is a necessity. In addition—witness *Sex and the City*—you're supposed to be part of a group of close-knit cronies who hang out together and know the intricate workings of one another's lives. But when you turn off the tube and look at how real people live, it's rarely this clear-cut.

For one thing, ours is an increasingly migratory society. If you're living in a city far from where you grew up or went to college, it can take a long time to create strong friendships. And if your job or your spouse's job calls for frequent moves, you have to learn to stay close to people you don't see often, as well as learn to make new friends quickly. Non-geographic life transitions change the friendship picture too. Getting married makes it harder to relate to your single friends. When you have a baby, you want to spend time with other moms. (And your childless buddies can't understand why you won't just get a sitter at the drop of some social hat.) People who are divorced or widowed find it hard not to feel like a third wheel in a world of twosomes. Even a career change makes it more difficult to maintain friendships with people with whom you once found common ground in shop talk.

There's also a self-knowledge piece here. Although we are a gregarious species, some of us are markedly more gregarious than others. At one end of the spectrum are those who find people fascinating, who eagerly talk with whomever is in the next seat on the plane, and who look around at concerts and sporting events thinking, "I would so love to hear all these people's stories." At the other extreme are those wearing headphones in lieu of a sandwich board that reads "LEAVE ME ALONE."

Gender generalizations have exceptions right and left, but recent research does suggest that platonic friendship is more of a need for women than for men. Landmark work done at UCLA suggests that women respond to stress not only by the standard "fight or flight" mechanism but by "tending and befriending"—caring for children and gathering with other women. Even so, some women—and some people in general—simply need more friends to feel safe and balanced than others do.

I'm pretty convivial, yet I've tended to attract men into my life who are—well, gosh, "hermits" is an extreme term, so let's just say "self-contained." My husband is very close to his family, but friends aren't a high priority. When my friend

Maggie came over for dinner and tried to make the point that New Yorkers don't champion diversity as much as we think we do, she asked William: "So who are your friends?" She was banking on his naming a dozen other white, Anglo-Saxon, male professionals. Instead, he replied, "I don't have any friends. I only know the people Victoria brings over here."

Now, that wasn't quite true. Upon prodding, he was able to come up with half a dozen names. Only Carlos (there's one point for the New-Yorkers-really-do-believe-in-diversity theory) is local, though, and Ted lives in Switzerland. William asked me later, "Do you think there's something wrong with me that I don't have more friends?" I said, "Do you want more friends?" He said he didn't, and I told him I probably had enough for both of us.

So, before you judge your quantity of sidekicks as if this were eighth grade and popularity a critical numbers game, ascertain if you're happy with the number of friends and the depth of the friendships you have now. If you are, no problem. If you want more profound friendships, you'll need to be willing to invest time in casual friends who have the potential to become close ones. If you'd like more friends, there are ways to meet people—get out, talk to strangers, take classes, join organizations—and to make the meetings more fruitful, as evidenced in the following ten tips from speaker and networking expert Olivia Fox (www.askolivia.com):

Ten Tips for Becoming Irresistible

1. *Put yourself in the other person's shoes.* He'll feel completely understood when you try to see everything from his perspective.

2. *Be really, truly interested in this person.* To quote Dale Carnegie: "You can make more friends in two months by becoming truly interested in other people than you can in two years by trying to get other people interested in you."

3. *Listen far more than you talk.* The longer you keep the spotlight on the other person, the more delightful he or she will find you.

4. *Smile!*

5. *Increase your level of eye contact.* This will send phenylethylamine (which scientists have called the love hormone) gushing through your veins, increasing interest on the part of both participants.

6. *Synchronize your body language with theirs.* Subtly (if you overdo this, it could backfire) assume the same postures, head tilt, facial expressions, and voice tone as the man or woman you're with. This will create a sense of, "How nice: we're just alike."

7. *Adopt a "What can I do for you?" mindset.*

8. *Be positive and enthusiastic.*

9. *Make the other person feel good about herself.* Admire and praise what you are truly impressed by. To be believable, be specific in your compliments.

10. *Quit worrying about what you just said, wish you hadn't said, or are going to say next.* In the end, people remember not what was said, but rather the emotional imprint of the conversation, how it *felt* to be talking with you.

These suggestions are as useful for relating to the friends, family, and business associates you already have as they are in the ice-breaking stages of meeting new people. Once someone is in your circle and your address book, don't let him or her languish there. Keep in touch. Short personal e-mails (as opposed to sappy forwards, unsolicited jokes, and your newsletter they didn't sign up for) are fine, and an actual note on real paper adds a touch of class. (When I'm going through a really organized period, I keep nice Crane's postcards, already stamped, in my purse so I can write a note while waiting for an appointment or a train.) Keeping track of birthdays is good, and remembering people when they least expect it is even better. You can send a card to acknowledge the anniversary of a friend's sobriety in AA, drop off a canine treat to acknowledge the adoption of a dog, or show up with a little gift to celebrate it's-one-month-after-the-breakup-and-you're-still-standing.

Getting into the habit of answering the phone only when you really do have time to talk keeps you from seeming perpetually crazy-busy and only concerned with your own goings-on. Suggesting unexpected outings (climbing a rock wall, taking a walking tour, or meeting for breakfast instead of the de rigueur dinner or lunch) will add to your reputation for being innovative and fun. And being available for friends when they need you will move you out of the fair-weather category into being a friend for all seasons.

Once you win all these friends, of course, you do have to put up with people. We are a complex lot, and we can be exasperating: we come in all types; we're dripping with beliefs and assumptions; and our moods can go from bitter to buoyant in less time than it takes those around us to make the shift. And yet we're good medicine for loneliness. To keep a friendship functional, set whatever boundaries you need to and communicate these clearly. It's a pity to have a friendship collapse because one person crossed over a line only the other knew was there. Go easy on your friends—they're likely to be hard on themselves; most of us are—but be honest too. Friends are one another's mirrors, and one another's teachers.

Take an Action

Do something special for a friend today. This can be a new friend—even someone who right now is just a potential one—or a tried-and-true friend who's been through the thick of it with you.

Chapter 38

ENTERTAIN, DAHLING

Lonely loves it when you sit around waiting for the phone to ring and can't bear it when you decide to have people over. There's a full catalog of excuses to draw from for not doing this: "I'm too busy.... My place is too small (or not nice enough).... I don't want to spend the money.... My friends would rather go out.... I'd have to clean up afterward.... My boyfriend doesn't like parties.... Somebody might smoke/get drunk/spill something/break something/be allergic to the parakeet.... I don't know what to serve or what to wear or whom to invite.... What if I go to all that trouble and people don't have a good time?" It's enough to keep you from letting the cable guy in.

And yet, what could be more delightful than surrounding yourself with handpicked people? Much of the time we're with the coworkers, neighbors, and strangers whose paths cross ours merely by happenstance. When you invite people over, though, they can be the ones you most want to spend time with. This is the case whether you're having a full-fledged party or a casual dinner for four (or five, the perfect number for a social meal, according to the ancient Greeks, who believed that with five the conversation flows smoothly and no one is left out).

There are so many ways to gather people together: wine and cheese after work, a potluck dinner Friday night, a backyard barbecue on the weekend. You can plan a gathering around something on TV—having friends over to watch the Oscars or the Super Bowl or the season finale of a show all of you follow. You might have a gathering to toast a friend who's gotten engaged or promoted or who's performed some act of bravery or moxie that deserves recognition. You may wish to celebrate holidays you wouldn't ordinarily think of—Chinese New Year, the equinox or solstice that will usher in the next new season, or the birthday of somebody famous.

When Adair was little, we started celebrating Mozart's birthday. It comes on a generally dismal day in late January (the 27th) when an Austrian-inspired dinner and a sheet cake decorated with a treble clef and music notes can assuage the winter blahs. Renting *Amadeus* makes an evening of it. A few days after we did this the first time, I heard my daughter, then seven, ask a little friend what he'd done for Mozart's birthday. I loved that to her it took only one celebration to invent a holiday. That's really all it has to take for any of us.

My entertaining mentor is the writer and storyteller Deborah Shouse, who celebrates holidays like March 4th (when you're supposed to, uh-huh, march forth into the rest of your year, the rest of your life). She also frequently gives theme parties, which have achieved local renown. When you show up for one of Deborah's soirées, it's often with a pre-assignment such as "Bring something of use or value that you're ready to pass on." A table is set with these items, rather like a collective tag sale, but upscale (she did say "of use or value") and without the tags. After dinner (always potluck: Deborah is a master entertainer who has no interest in cooking), one guest at a time goes to the table and claims a gift, telling the group why he or she chose the particular item. At one of these gatherings, I selected a mother-of-pearl statue of a yellow cat. My cat Albert, straw-colored and much beloved, had passed away a few days earlier. Although I'm not the bric-a-brac type, I was meant to have that cat. Other people shared similar serendipities.

If you're not used to having people over, a great way to activate your entertaining aptitude is to host a salon. Because this is a cross between a party and a meeting, you can schedule it for midafternoon or after dinner and avoid the whole issue of serving food. The idea of a salon is to discuss an issue, explore a topic, do a project, or read a book or article and talk about it. It can be a onetime event—for instance, gathering four or five friends to make vision-maps (see chapter 27)—or a series, such as five every-other-week gatherings to discuss the five sections of this book and the progress everyone is making in getting past fat, broke & lonely.

When you're ready to bring a meal into your repertoire, invite one person or one couple for dinner. If you don't want to cook, hire a caterer or order a pizza, in keeping with your budget and your inclination. This is just a way to get your entertaining land legs. Expand from there. Nobody is going to run a white glove along your baseboards checking for dust, and a review of the meal will not appear in tomorrow's food section. Opening your home to people you like is simply a way to add more joy to your life and more life to your house or apartment.

Sure, your friends might bring flowers or a candle or a bottle of wine, but what they'll really leave behind is the energy of the time you shared. Realtors (as well as psychics) will tell you that houses *feel* happy or sad, energized or weary, based on what's gone on in them over the years. Every time you open your doors to people who bring in laughter and affection, you get to keep some of it after they go, both in memory and in the ethers of the place where you live. Then, when you come in from work to your single-girl flat, or to the house where your kids used to make a ruckus but they're grown up and gone now, there will be a lightness there that loneliness assiduously avoids. But you'll like it. Chances are it will spur you on to plan another party.

Take an Action

If you never entertain, just get another human being or two into your home. If you do entertain sometimes, set a date for your next get-together. Try something different from your usual. Above all, make it a point to have fun. If you do, chances are your guests will too.

Chapter 39

IT'S NOT ALWAYS ABOUT YOU

You call it quits with lonely and come to grips with life the instant you realize that it's not always about you. This can happen at sixteen or sixty, the moment you know without question that the best way to get out of yourself, your worries, and your loneliness is to make someone else's day. This does not in any way diminish your magnificence or the need to take exquisite care of yourself. It's simply opening up to the paradox that your life becomes richer when you see that it's not always about you—your looks, your success, your desires. That's when you'll want to put your time, heart, and sweat where they can do some good.

It's a fact: somebody out there needs you. I don't know if it's an elder in a nursing home, a child in the foster system, a family uprooted by a natural disaster, or your mom who really loves you even though you guys don't talk. But I know without even having met you that somebody needs your love, your proficiency at algebra, or your skill with a hammer.

Getting out of yourself and transforming somebody else's world can be a major undertaking—six months of work in a developing country, say—or a momentary kindness like walking lost tourists back to their hotel instead of just pointing the way. (My friend Heather did this with a very old, nearly blind Asian man who spoke only a few words of English. After some trial and quite a bit of error, she delivered him to his destination, where she was informed that her charge was a revered Tibetan *rinpoche* and that she would be fortunate indeed to be kept in his prayers.)

One way to get out of yourself and become part of something wonderful is through formal volunteering. Volunteer opportunities all over America are listed at www.volunteermatch.org, and some ask for a surprisingly small time commitment. Another website, www.idealist.org, has postings for volunteers needed both in the United States and overseas, as well as some full-time paying jobs. You can also simply say yes to extemporaneous opportunities to be a force for good. Whom you help doesn't matter. That you help matters a lot.

Follow your own leanings when you look for ways to make things better—one kind act at a time. My daughter, Adair, has always loved anybody with four paws and even as a child rescued strays and spoke out for animals. After she got married and found herself overwhelmed with the pressures of pursuing an acting career in New York City, holding down a day job, and maintaining an apartment, she realized that walking her two dogs, even though it was one more item on the to-do list, was often a high point of her day.

"It's so therapeutic," she says. "Even though I hate going out in the winter when it's cold, it's just for them. Doing something purely for somebody else makes me feel good. And they never care how I look or what I wear." Her dog-walking epiphany was so pronounced that she signed on as a volunteer walker for homeless canines waiting for a human of their very own. Adair still has auditions and callbacks and classes and shows, a mortgage to share and a living to make. The time she spends with her dogs and the orphans in their "You Can Adopt Me" jackets, however, seems to extend her day rather than intrude on it. Maybe that's because sixty minutes of being fully alive is quite different from an hour of the ordinary.

As you come to understand that it's not always about you, understand, too, that each of us is uniquely wired. Some people are natural do-gooders. They thrive on helping. Many gravitate to careers such as nursing or psychotherapy that let them help people from here to retirement. Others adopt a houseful of special-needs children, or there's an apron with their name on it at the soup kitchen. If this sounds to you like an alien way of life, it's just not your path. You can still help, but in a way that doesn't make you feel like it's Halloween and you're going as Florence Nightingale.

Give what you have. Teach what you know. Trust your instincts. When you read or hear about a situation and it particularly speaks to you, follow up. There is so much suffering in the world that we become largely immune to it just to go on functioning. When the plight of one person or one place bypasses this immune response and goes straight to your soul, chances are that's your cause. One can be enough.

When you take action on something that speaks to you in this way, whether as a lifetime commitment or a one-day assignment, you will meet people who share your spiritual genes. They showed up at the same time and the same place as you because you both felt moved to be there. There's no way of predicting where you'll meet someone who'll still be in your life after your grandchildren grow up, but this is as good a place as any and far better than most.

Meanwhile, be useful when you can be useful and shine your light every chance you get, even—and perhaps especially—for those who don't seem able to give you anything in return. Sherry—my action partner that you met earlier—did this between one station and the next on a crowded subway. She became aware of hubbub on the train-car as people edged away from the middle, all trying to avoid a dirty homeless man whose midsummer stench was overpowering. He sat alone on the bench, looking forlornly at the scores of repulsed straphangers and clutching his one earthly good: a dented box of Cheerios.

As the train approached her stop, Sherry gave the man a sincere smile and wished him a good day. He said, "Thank you. You're the first person who's spoken to me in a long time." It was the moment of eye contact that Sherry says she will long remember. "I felt that my heart had really met his. Just before that, I'd been caught up in myself and my stuff. But at that moment, I got to be present to someone else. I spoke to him first, but he gave me the gift."

Take an Action

Find a way to do some serious good in the world. Giving money is fine, but today's action calls for giving of yourself. Help is needed all around you. Try holding the door, giving somebody a hand with their bags, taking the time to provide directions to that perplexed-looking couple with the map. You can also connect with a charity or sign up to volunteer somewhere. It may not feel like your ultimate philanthropic calling, but it will do till that shows up.

Chapter 40

CHARISMA 101

You are already in possession of a powerful anti-lonely resource: the people in your life right now. You can see this by bringing to mind everyone in your personal sphere you're really glad to have there. Jot down their first names and look at the list. Size doesn't matter. Quality does. You have just documented the existence of the men, women, children, and golden retrievers you have attracted into your life. (In a metaphysical sense, you even "attracted" your parents and grandparents through magnetism at the soul level.) Congratulations. You've done well. And you've illustrated for yourself the law of attraction at work.

It is your personal magnetism that draws people and experiences into your world. We all know about physical attraction: you see a great-looking stranger on a bus, and your body gears up for sex and your mind for a life together. But magnetism goes so much further. It's that first impression that makes you feel that a new acquaintance could become a friend, or that a particular candidate would make a good leader.

When personal magnetism is extraordinary, we call it charisma. Derived from the Greek *kharis*, "divine favor," charisma was seen by the ancients as a gift from the gods. But its qualities—physical vigor, confidence, the ability to inspire others—can be developed by anyone who wants them enough. That would be you, since you've decided to make the break with fat, broke & lonely.

Obviously, if you want to do something huge—run for the Senate, raise $50 million to help cure something, host a talk show on national TV—you'll need some serious charisma: a golden-girl persona, oratorical prowess, near-total recall of faces, names, and facts, and a preternatural penchant for witty repartee. Fine. If that's the desire of your heart, that's what you have to do. Get yourself to Toastmasters and hire a media coach. If you're looking instead for a bliss-kissed life with a nice guy and a host of friends who won't let you down, you can increase your ability to attract more of what you want with less rehearsing and fewer tied-up evenings. Whatever you desire, your charisma—your own personal magnetism—draws to you. Here are some ways to increase it, regardless of what—or whom—you're looking to attract:

- *Glow with good health*. Feng shui experts say that a vibrantly healthy plant increases the sense of well-being in a home or office. A vibrantly healthy *person* does this in spades. Physical vitality can give sex appeal to someone who isn't particularly handsome or beautiful, and just being around this degree of vigor makes mere bystanders feel better. Get it for yourself by seeing yourself in the glow of health and supporting the vision by eating food with its life force intact, exercising as if you actually wanted to, and treating your body as a temple, even before your temple has a flat stomach.

- *Emanate enthusiasm.* As with charisma, we can thank the Greeks for enthusiasm, the word anyway, coming as it does from *en theos,* "with God." I think of enthusiasm as having a fire inside that keeps you pumped and passionate and committed. Everything that keeps your energy up—getting enough sleep, getting out in the world and being part of things, keeping your focus on what you want while being grateful for what you have—keeps your enthusiasm up too. And because nobody can be enthusiastic nonstop, have positive people around you to carry the torch when you're having trouble keeping yours lit.

- *Speak sincerely.* Phonies are as transparent as the wrapping on your sandwich. If there's conviction behind your words, the people who need to hear them will listen.

- *Be interested in just about everything.* His siblings used to refer to my younger stepson, James, as "the Discovery Channel" because he was so interested in finding out about everything. He still is, and it's a most endearing quality. When you know a lot about a lot of things, you can talk with anyone and make that person feel at ease. The idea is not to trump the *Jeopardy* contestants every night but to have a wide enough range of interests that other people don't feel they have to be experts in your business or your hobby to have a fascinating conversation with you. It's also easier to think on your feet when your internal search engine has plenty to draw from.

- *Keep an upbeat attitude.* If you look at how things are, it's easy to get discouraged, and that wreaks havoc with your charisma. You may need to take a few hours or a day to focus on a problem, wrestle with a demon, or otherwise get down and dirty with the tough stuff. If that's the case, go somewhere, close the door, and focus, wrestle, or get down. When you've done it, even if the dilemma at hand is not fully solved, come out certain that it will be.

- *Become the person you want to be to attract the person (or people) you want to attract.* This ought to be clear as day, but we miss it all the time: we attract people and experiences that are in keeping with our personal frequency. "I'm looking for a financially stable man" sounds smart, but if you're in debt up to your armpits and you spend every weekend at the racetrack, he's not looking for you. After a series of flubbed relationships, a friend of mine wrote down every quality she wanted in a boyfriend and *then proceeded to develop those very attributes in herself.* It took several months, but she met someone with the character traits she was looking for (he's also cute, for what that's worth), and they've been together successfully for six years.

- *Cultivate clear boundaries.* Being liked is great; being stalked isn't. As you boost your charisma, strengthen at the same time the parameters that delineate your personal space. I once saw Lauren Bacall in the Oak Bar at the Plaza Hotel. She was pure movie-star presence, exquisitely turned out, politely focused on her companion, totally gracious in her demeanor, and *no one would have dared go near her.* Her boundaries were as real as if they'd been built of concrete. You can have protective boundaries like that too, deciding how much of yourself to give, when, and to whom. It's not selfish. It's self-preservation.

- *Plug into a power source that won't give out.* Charisma is power coming through a person. We don't generate it; we channel it. Remember "divine favor"? Maybe those Greeks weren't so far off. Human power, even at its best, is limited. Plug into the unlimited and there's nothing you can't do.

Take an Action

First, envision yourself as a charismatic person, one possessing powerful charm. Then, take one of the preceding steps toward developing your own charismatic qualities. Try it for three days and you will feel the difference.

Part Five

HOOKING UP WITH
THE LIFE OF YOUR DREAMS

You came to this planet to be remarkable.
You do that by being yourself, using your gifts,
and shining your light.

It is a great day when you know that, as long as you keep doing what you're doing and thinking how you're thinking, fat, broke, lonely, and the agonizing part of the emptiness that invited them in at the start can be out of your life for good. This is not the end, however: it's the beginning. Avoiding what you don't want is just the prerequisite. The life of your dreams is the course you signed up for.

You came to this planet to be remarkable. This doesn't necessarily mean stretching your fifteen minutes of fame to twenty-five, or making a tsunami-sized splash in the world, but it might. The only limits to what you can do are the constraints of time, space, and physics. When we limit ourselves more than that—and we're all guilty of it—we short-circuit destiny. It's your obligation to swing for the fences. Whether or not you make the home run is beside the point.

To hook up with the life of your dreams, it is essential, first, to know what your dreams are. To go forward, you'll have to look fear in the face and walk right through it. You'll need to become crystal clear about who you are and what you stand for, and put into practice some simple but powerful techniques that people who are living the life of their dreams already know about. You'll be asked to glimpse who you really are and what you're connected to. This is a challenging and demanding process, and because it is, I wouldn't count on its becoming a trend anytime soon. But if you're up for it, you won't just steer clear of fat, broke & lonely: you'll be in for the adventure of a lifetime.

Chapter 41

YA GOTTA HAVE A DREAM

There ought to be a Society for the Prevention of Cruelty to Dreams, the way they're ignored and kicked around and tossed aside. We say terrible things about them: "Yeah, I wanted to go to Harvard, but that was just stupid." We even defame them to the next generation: "You're never going to be [on Broadway, in the NHL, on a Fashion Week runway], so cut out the [singing, skating, walking around with a book on your head]." Dreams that can make it through all that have to be remarkably resilient. Remarkably, some are.

The reason we're so hard on dreams is that we're trying to shield ourselves and those we care about from the disappointment of a dream that doesn't materialize. But if you go for it, you succeed just for starting. Sure, it'll hurt if you don't get the part or the job, but you'll always know you were there giving it your best shot. That puts texture in your life and gives you stories to tell your grandchildren.

History is filled with luminaries who lost out on one dream only to embrace another. Audrey Hepburn trained to be a

ballerina. Several of Milton Hershey's businesses went bank-
rupt before he came up with the five-cent chocolate bar. Because Levi and Strauss weren't selling enough tents to miners,
they turned to durable clothing, and that's the reason you're
wearing jeans.

Even though the dream that comes true may not be the
one you start out with, you have to aim now for the one
you've got. If it morphs or shifts or detours, you can deal with
that, but to give up on it prematurely means you lose twice:
this dream bites the dust, and it doesn't get the opportunity to
turn into something else.

Although theoretically possible, having a dream that's just
plum nuts is rare. When I speak before large groups of women,
I ask if anybody has as her dream to become an Olympic
gymnast. No one has ever raised her hand. Obviously, if
you're over twelve, that would be a ridiculous dream, *and we
don't have ridiculous dreams.* The dreams you are carrying around
this minute are real, and there is a basis for them. Otherwise,
you'd have different ones.

Don't be daunted by the size of your dream. It may seem
enormous only because it's the one you happen to want. Let's
say you've set your sights on becoming a CEO. Admittedly,
getting there will take some doing, but for me, and plenty of
other people, it sounds less like a big dream than a big pain. If
you want it, though, and you're scaring yourself because it
seems so huge and so desirable, think of all of us who wouldn't
take the job at any salary. That should put it in perspective:
you have this particular dream because it's possible for you to
achieve it and excel at it. Once you get that piece, you have
to transform the CEO thing from an idea in your head into a

sign on your door. That means work—on the metaphysical level and the megaphysical level.

The metaphysical work is what you do spiritually to help create your reality. We've talked about meditation (chapter 9), using positive language (chapter 7), and visualization and vision-maps (chapter 27). If you are serious about this dream of yours, involve every sense you're equipped with. When moving to New York was a dream of mine—and believe me, it looked like an impossible one—I heard Dr. Jean Houston, author of *A Passion for the Possible,* speak in Kansas City. She led her listeners through an exercise of bringing our dreams into being by employing all our senses. In that experience, I *heard* the sirens and traffic of Manhattan. I *smelled* the sweetness of flowers at a corner market and the stench of a Canal Street fish market. I *felt* my arm stretch to hail a taxi, then reach out to open the door. As I slipped inside the imaginary cab, I took a crusty bagel out of a deli bag and *tasted* the bland satisfaction of the doughy delicacy. It was the closest I'd ever been to New York without changing time zones.

The power of that was such that I kept it up. Along with positive thinking and glancing daily at a skyscraper-studded vision-map, I started listening to Broadway show tunes and actually eating bagels, and I did this you're-there-already exercise three or four times a week. Within a year, my area code was 212.

But there is the other piece: the megaphysical work. That encompasses the physical and mental rigors you have to go through to give substance, dimension, and here-and-now reality to something that has been formless. While the metaphysical work lays the foundation, the megaphysical work builds the structure. In my New York example, I did the work required to get a book contract before the move; I collected a long list of networking contacts; and I made an Arthurian pre-trip in search of that elusive grail, an affordable sublet. Whatever your dream, it's going to demand some exertion. You may have to go back to school. Get in the best shape of your life. Learn Arabic or Mandarin. Audition 2,416 times. Or go through fertility treatments, have them fail, and find yourself on the other side of the world holding your baby, clutching your dream.

Don't be afraid of the effort. You don't have to do it all today, but you do have to do today's share. Sometimes it won't seem fair. You could be working two jobs to get your degree while everybody else seems to have either a full scholarship or rich parents. You might have to move to a strange city or even a strange country, and then discover when you arrive that the place is full of people who want just what you do except that they were born there and know the ropes. You may have to overcome the negativity and resistance of family and friends, while someone else gets a rousing send-off and nonstop support. Of course it sucks. But you can focus either on that or on knocking down the nearest barrier that stands between you and your dream.

Don't get hung up on other people's advantages. Everyone has advantages, including you. What have you got? Money, education, and social position? Good looks, good health, and exceptional talent? Linguistic ability and people skills? Shrewdness and wit? A Ph.D. in street smarts? Your advantages are yours to exploit in the service of your dream. In other words, if your father owns the company you want to work for, good for you. If he doesn't, you've got your MBA, your published thesis, and your ability to remember verbatim everything anybody says for the rest of your natural life. Will the road be easier for Daddy's little girl? Maybe, maybe not. It's none of your business. You only have to do the work (metaphysical and megaphysical) and bring your best self to the office.

Take an Action

This one is a three-parter:

1. Write down what your dream is. If you don't know yet, just write until it shows up.

2. Take two actions, one metaphysical and one mega-physical, to move you toward your dream.

3. List the dream-catching advantages you have right now. Read them over and get comfortable with the idea of using them.

Chapter 42

FULL FRONTAL FEARLESS

We think we're afraid of being fat, broke, lonely, and the rest. Not exactly: we're afraid—terrified, in fact—of feeling. We respond with filler behaviors (eating, spending, setting our cap for a guy who's said eleven times he's gay) to avoid feeling empty, afraid, alone, or unsure of ourselves. But here's the catch: feelings—every gnawing, nagging sensation—are frightening only until you've felt them. After that, they turn to dust and blow away. Then you understand that you were never really dealing with pizzas, paychecks, and pals (or lack of them). It was all about feelings, some of them so old they don't even know disco died.

Your task going forward is to stay put and stay present, rather than try to delete uncomfortable feelings like unread spam. It's scarier than anything the people on *Fear Factor* will ever come up with: sitting with feelings and not canceling them out with a filler behavior of any stripe. The greats all did it: Gautama sat with his unknowing long enough to arise as the Buddha (a word that translates as "one who woke up").

Jesus sparred in the wilderness with Satan (symbolic, according to some theologians, of unchecked ego) and came out the Christ (translation: "anointed one"). Every day ordinary folks sit without ordering the drink, eating the brownie, or buying the shoes. And they walk away free.

When people go to empowerment camps or self-realization seminars where they break blocks of wood and walk on hot coals, it's for the purpose of facing and overcoming a fear straight on. Thundering music enlivens the board-breaking, shamanic drumming facilitates the fire-walk, and cheering co-campers spur confidence throughout. It's a dramatic experience that becomes a vivid memory, one the participants can draw on even years later. An experience like this is an initiatory rite, and I highly recommend that you partake of a cliff-climbing, rapids-rafting, sky-diving, wilderness-survival, simulated-mugging, or related scenario if you can. There are, however, plenty of opportunities to prove yourself in regular life too, although the music is more likely to be Muzak and chances are there won't be anybody cheering. That makes a real-life freefall even more of a challenge, and walking away unscathed even more of a victory.

There are all sorts of scary things to meet and overcome daily. The worst ones, barring actual tragedies and disasters, are those on your private list: authority figures ... speaking in public ... the annual checkup ... saying something dumb ... legal-looking envelopes from creditors, lawyers, or the IRS. Even though someone else may have no problem whatsoever with those particular people or situations, they leave you shivering in your trendy lace-up boots. If you were able to watch a movie of your entire life, you could probably pinpoint the exact moment when that family of circumstances first shifted from neutral into petrifying, but even with that information, you'd still have to deal with your checkup this afternoon and the envelope in your mailbox tonight. The way out of any of it—and you already know this—is through.

It helps to understand that fear, its fraternal twin shame, and their first cousin guilt—the feelings we most abhor—are standard operating equipment for *homo sapiens*. You're not going to eradicate them, so you may as well save your breath. The fear we're so afraid of is simply a biochemical reaction. It's measurable. Your heart rate quickens, your adrenal glands release adrenaline, your mouth gets dry, and you may sweat right through your roll-on. Your response to a job interview can be the same fight-or-flight reaction with which our Stone Age ancestors met a full-scale attack from a mastodon, but since you can't punch the HR person or run very far in your Jimmy Choos, you sit and stew in your own stress hormones.

"I teach people to face fear, understand it, accept that it's there, and change their relationship with it," says Thom Rutledge, psychotherapist and author of *Embracing Fear*. "You have to understand that fear is a bully that lives in your head. It's useless, destructive, neurotic, and you're going to disagree with it. The recovery position is 'I see you, I hear you, I disagree with you.' You don't get rid of fear, but you stop being controlled by it." Rutledge suggests "pronoun therapy." Instead of saying, "I'm scared out of my wits; I'm so going to screw this up," switch to the second-person pronoun: "You're scared spitless; you're so going to screw this up." That clarifies that the fear is talking, not you, and you can talk back.

You can also talk with your friends, call on your faith, and whistle in the pitch-dark if you have to. When you find a fear-facing technique that works for you, use it. Maybe you're good at breaking down your fears: in little pieces, they're far less intimidating. Or you might play the worst-case-scenario game and see what's the worst that could happen. Often we generate a life-or-death amount of fear for a this-could-be-slightly-unpleasant circumstance. If a fear is causing trouble in your actual life—you're afraid of being alone, for example, so you stay in a destructive relationship—make dealing with that fear a priority. Finally, don't let other people plant fears in your head. Whether it's your mom who thinks you ought to be married or the local newscaster who's going to tell you about the danger lurking in your garden hose, you have enough going on with the fears you already have on file. Accept no further donations.

You walk through a midsized fear ("I have to talk to my boss's boss") or a monumental one ("I go to court on Friday and could lose my apartment") the same way—steadily, one step at a time. Even when you're afraid and showing tender mercies to yourself is totally called for, the basic rules don't change. It's still okay to go out for a nice dinner with some-one who makes you laugh; it's still not okay to hole up with a foot-long chili-cheese dog and a box of chocolates. It's okay to buy yourself a gift you can pay for; it's not okay to buy one you can't. It's okay to hold someone's hand, and in fact you ought to, but it's not okay to sleep with a stranger just because you're scared.

When you've sat with the feelings and walked through the fear, you are a new, or at least re-newed, person. Stronger. Braver. Calmer. Gutsier. And more alive than you've ever been.

Take an Action

Make a list of everything you're afraid of. Share it with your action partner or another trusted friend. Work from the inside out, asking your Higher Power for help in defusing these fears. Then destroy your list in some histrionic fashion. Burn it (safely, of course), or shred it, or tear it into little pieces and toss them off a skyscraper or into a moving stream. This will not turn you into an intrepid super-hero, but if you put some genuine intention into your action, it will help disarm some of the fright-bullies.

Chapter 43

PUT TOGETHER YOUR DREAM TEAM

The next time you watch a movie, sit through all the credits. It's mind-boggling that it takes so many people to produce two hours of entertainment, but it does. Almost everything in existence got here by group effort, and your dream will come into being that way too. I hope that by now you have an action partner: one compatible person who has both your best interest and her own at heart. Let's up the ante now and get you a whole dream team.

The starting point, your core dream team, is a dedicated group of people committed to their own progress and to holding a vision of success for one another. Their motto: "You can do anything you set your mind to, and we're going to make sure you don't forget it." This kind of supportive circle has been called a *mastermind alliance.* Like the proverbial superiority of two heads to one, four or five or six minds form a mastermind in which each individual's information and experience are multiplied into exponential levels of know-how, and each individual's contacts lead to diminishing degrees of separation.

For a mastermind group to do all it can for all its members, everyone has to make it a priority. Odds are that a few people won't. For this reason, start with a large enough base that your group can lose a couple of members and not miss them. (Eight is a good number: half could bail and you'd still have a team.) Put out feelers among your friends and colleagues for people who would like to be part of such an alliance. Choose carefully. It's your dream we're working on here. Do you want a group that's single-gender or coed? Is it important that everyone work in your industry or have small children or be about your age? If you join an existing group, these questions will have already been answered. If you start a group, it can be customized to your specifications. Watch out for taking on the role of leader, though. All responsibilities should be shared so that everyone contributes and benefits equally.

Once it's been organized, the group needs to gather in real time and space on a regular basis—maybe once a week for breakfast or twice a month on a weekday evening, whatever seems right. When you meet, plan to go around the circle and give everyone a chance to talk without interruption for an allotted period—three minutes maybe, or five (have someone keep time). After the initial go-round, open it up so people can share information and offer suggestions as called for. The only ground rule—and this one is sacrosanct—is that criticism is not allowed. Saying, "Have you ever considered looking at it this way?" is fine. "That's the most idiotic idea I've ever heard" isn't.

Jealousy—do you notice how "lousy" is such a big part of that word?— will kill a dream team (and heaven knows, it's killed its share of dreams). Envy is a diabolical emotion because it says that there isn't enough to go around. This sets up a worldview of a stingy universe, and if that's where you think you live, that's where they'll send your mail. Even if everybody in the group gets promoted, elected, married, pregnant, and named "Person of the Year" before you, you have to rejoice in their joy. Know that it's contagious and that if you weren't doing a whole lot right as a group, these delights wouldn't be befalling its members. Your unfolding dreams are on their way. For now, it's imperative that you learn to uncork the champagne for those whose dreams came in on the express train.

Once these basic principles of camaraderie are established, the group belongs to those who comprise it. Yours might study books about business or spirituality or something else. You might divide up the year so that each of your half-dozen members gets two full months when the major efforts of the group are on her behalf. You could bring in an expert to teach everybody Photoshop or feng shui. However you set things up, the primary reason you're together is to be one another's dream team, one that will stop at nothing to get the heart's desire of each person up and running.

Your dream may call for significant others in addition to your mastermind alliance and your action partner. If you're stuck because of old stuff, you may need to see a qualified therapist (or see one again if you've been there, done that, and you're still stuck). Your dream may be waiting in the wings until you get educated in a certain area or perfect a

certain skill. The teacher or mentor who'll help you there becomes part of your dream team even if you never tell her
you've got one. Maybe you just need a cheerleader, someone
with whom you have no emotional involvement and whose
job it is to be sure you get from where you are to where you
want to be as expeditiously as possible. If this sounds good,
you may want to look into hiring a life coach who's been
trained to help carve out of your life all that isn't conducive to
your dream, the way Michelangelo carved from the stone all
that wasn't David.

When you think of your everyday life as part and parcel of
the remarkable life you're creating, everyone who lends a
hand takes on honorary dream-team status. The guy who
does your taxes, because numbers make you cross-eyed, and
the one who presses your shirts, because you need that time
for night classes, are both part of it. When you come to see
the vital roles that a host of people play in helping birth your
dream, you'll appreciate them more—and you already know
what appreciation will get you.

Take an Action

Take the initial steps toward establishing your mastermind
circle. Send around an e-mail to people you think might be
interested. Plan the first meeting and know that the faces
you see around that table will be the ones that are supposed to be there.

Chapter 44

LIGHT UP YOUR LOOK

We live in an appearance-oriented time and place. Women have long been judged by how they look, and men are increasingly feeling the pressure as well. Looking hot (or, when you're past the age of hot, looking attractive and younger than your driver's license says you ought to) has become a hoop through which we're all supposed to jump in order to achieve success and happiness. This is overblown and off base. People who neglect who they are to focus on how they appear are like snazzy cars, all spiffed and polished, with no engines under their shimmering hoods.

There's a fine line here, though. Even as the media urges us to overdo in the looking-good arena, many people underdo—perhaps in response to all the coercion from the other side. Although you have every right to look however you like, first impressions do impress, for good or ill. If you can light up a room via the combination of a loving spirit and knockout mascara, people remember that. Getting from here to the life of your dreams doesn't call for looking like a model or a pageant princess, just showing the world your cleaned-up, cared-for self. And when you light up your look from the inside first, you won't worry nearly so much about encroaching birthdays or rebellious hair days.

Not long ago I was at a large gathering and noticed a young woman who was reasonably pretty but who had *presence* that was far more striking. She seemed to be illuminated from within in a way that made me want to get to know her and listen to every word she had to say. Later that day I ran into a guy I know who'd also been at this event. "Did you see that amazing woman?" he asked with no prompting from me. "She almost made me wish I was straight."

That the two of us responded as we did to a total stranger is anecdotal evidence that this inner-light business is not just the stuff of poetry and folklore. It is the very foundation of beauty and appeal. When you have it, you're beautiful regardless of your features. People start to see you as *enchanting* and *mesmerizing*. It's because they have inner light too, even if they've kept theirs under a bushel for years. When someone glimpses that light in another person, there's a warm sense of recognition—sort of like you get when you're in a strange city and see somebody in a sweatshirt from your college.

You know the tired weight-loss saw "Inside every fat person is a thin one trying to get out"? Well, inside all the hurried, harried, insecure humans who wonder what would happen if other people knew how clueless they really felt, there is this light, a reflection of the greater Light that got us here. Robert Browning called this truth and power inside us "the imprisoned splendor." Yours has been trying to get out since the first time you smiled. It will shine like the dickens when given half a chance. You give it that chance by, first, acknowledging its existence and then going out into the world dedicated to letting the Light do its thing.

Every time you express love, every time you do somebody a good turn without feeling resentful about it, you're shining your light. Every time you're excited about something, or laugh out loud, or feel that surge of hopefulness as if it wouldn't take much wind to get you airborne—that's the Light. Whenever you know that things will work out when that's not how they look, or you do something you don't want to with good faith and good humor, or you gaze at a sunset or a sycamore and get embarrassingly moved by the experience, your light is on.

Some people like to envision this luminescence residing within their body, within their heart. You can envision yours there when you meditate and anytime during the day when a little light could help things. Think of your heart, the vital center of your physical being, as also the center of your spiritual being while you're in this body. Just as blood is pumped by your physical heart, light flows from your spiritual heart, filling every part of you. And it isn't confined to your body: it surrounds you with peace and protection, so that fewer things get to you. Its reach extends to everyone you meet, giving the light in each of them a little jump-start.

The more you relate to and work with your inner light, the lovelier you'll appear—*and* the better you'll care for your outer being. You'll look stunning because you'll know you already are, not because you hope the right haircut and outfit will make you into something you believe deep down you're not.

Taking better care of your outer self doesn't necessarily mean wearing makeup every day (or ever, if you're not the makeup type). It does, however, mean giving your top-of-the-line shot to preparing for whatever is on tap that day, whether you'll be jogging around the track or walking down the aisle. When I don't care enough to do this—"I'm only going to a movie and it'll be dark"—I instantly time-travel back to the days of eating for a fix, not having any money, and not caring enough about anything. That's the worst kind of déjà vu. To stay on course, I don't need a $1,000 makeover every time I see daylight, but I do need to maintain a baseline of self-care and add to that as indicated. Everybody is going to have a different baseline, ranging from clean hair and sunblock to regularly scheduled appointments for brow-shaping, high-lights, seaweed wraps, and bikini waxing.

Nobody looks like those people on the red carpet every day. Even *they* don't look like that every day. But if you shine your light, believe in who you are, and take care of yourself on gloomy days as well as glorious ones, you'll be ready when the person or the opportunity you've been waiting for shows up. And that could happen when you least expect it.

Take an Action

For the next seven days, light up your look inside and out. First, acknowledge your Light within—the substance of your beauty—and then present your physical self to the world each day as if it did indeed house that Light. If you feel that you can't do the physical part without first getting your roots touched up, seeing the shoe repair guy, and sewing on several buttons, get these preliminaries out of the way ASAP so you can start on your week of living fabulously.

Chapter 45

ONE DAY A WEEK, UNPLUG AND RECONNECT

It makes sense, if you work five days a week, to take one of the others for errands and laundry and catching up. The seventh day, however, is your opportunity to unplug and reconnect. Even God rested, metaphorically at least, and we're supposed to rest too. If you're part of a religion that has specific Sabbath teachings, there's little question about what you are to do and not do on that day. The rest of us are apt to fill it like any other—with the labor and detritus of *doing*—when in fact every one of us could use a day to refresh, regroup, and put some punctuation between the week just past and the one that's coming.

To hook up with the life of your dreams, you need twenty-four hours a week for yourself and your spirit, exploration and play, family and friends, and all the important stuff there's never enough time for in "real life." This is the day that, if you're willing to take it, will pay you back with better health, greater clarity, and more energy all week long.

Setting one day aside like this is also a way to reset your personal clock. Not only do you get a lavishly lengthy Sunday or Saturday (or whatever day works for you), but you may find yourself less pressed for time the rest of the week. Remember when we talked about tithing and how the people who do it are convinced that giving 10 percent of their money results in their having more? Taking a day apart for personal and spiritual pursuits works the same way: people who do it find that they have more time.

On this day, it's helpful to unplug from the two most powerful external influences around: the computer and the TV. This is not because either one is inherently evil. I happen to think they're inherently remarkable, spiritual even, in their capacity to connect people and help us understand one another. On the downside, however, they focus your attention outward, away from your inner direction. Why not use them and enjoy them all week long, but for one day pull the plug? This is the day when you don't have to tend to e-mail or put up with background noise. It is your day apart, when your interior inklings and the desires of your heart are the sites to visit and the shows to watch. On your unplugged day, you get to focus on your own life.

Chicago writer Amy Gonigam, who has experimented with extended unplugged periods, says, "Twice I have disabled my Internet browser at home. I've had to reinstall it both times because I realized I can't live without it, but when I've trashed it, I've had such serenity. There were huge blocks of time to read and meditate. It's possible to sit down and pretend to check e-mail and spend hours on stuff that just doesn't matter." TV can be the same way. It's a terrific medium when you tune in to something moving or important, informative or funny, but clicking the remote as a reflex action gives away your power. When you unplug for a day, you get that power back—along with those "huge blocks of time."

In addition to taking a break from technology, you can use your personal sabbath for R&R (and R): rest, recreation, and reconnecting. Rest by setting aside, just for a day, your regular work, both the kind you bring home from the office and what they used to call "woman's work" that was "never done." (Now men and women are supposed to do it together, which is better, but it's still never done.) Taking a day of rest isn't some fanatical proclamation. Obviously, you have to take care of the basics. If your boss calls, you'll probably want to pick up. You can also make the bed and even pancakes unless you resent making either one or doing so detracts from your idea of a restful time-out. This could be the day you give your joints and muscles a break from working out, although you might opt to go to the gym with your guy or a gaggle of girlfriends just for the fun of it. Recreation, whatever re-creates *you*, is so very allowed.

There's a strong precedent for balancing the workweek with a day of serious play. When I was a tiny kid in a conservative part of the country, nearly all stores and businesses were closed on Sunday, and you couldn't buy a brandy even if it was to save somebody from hypothermia. It was, however, the biggest day of the week for recreational outlets—movies, live theater, museums, amusement parks, sporting events. They're still open. Get over there.

Finally, use this day for connecting with anything that gets short shrift during the week. Your hopes and dreams, for instance. Nature. Your inner self. Your painting or your novel.

It's the perfect day to get together with the friends who moved to the suburbs or to talk at length with your cousin who moved to Seattle. This is the day you can join Walt Whitman in saying, "I loaf and invite my soul," and see this luxurious loafing as a grand avocation.

With so much of our time prearranged for work and other commitments, it's oddly glorious to have one day that you can arrange to suit yourself. On my unplug-and-reconnect day, Sunday, William and I usually walk to church through Central Park and have lunch out after. The rest of the day is unique in the vastness of its options. My only "rules" are to stay (1) unplugged and (2) true to myself. (I guess "make this a fantastic day" is a kind of rule too, but it doesn't seem like one.)

If you think of it, a day is kind of like a gift card from Victoria's Secret. You can spend it on a black lace-up corset that isn't very comfortable but makes your true love happy. That's fine: it made somebody happy. But every now and then you have to trade that card in for the cozy pajamas or the soft cammy that would feel good next to your very own skin. One day out of every seven, this card's for you.

Take an Action

Choose a day of the week that fits your schedule and your sentiments and earmark it as the one you'll set aside to unplug and reconnect. This is your day to rest, have fun, and immerse yourself in the people and projects that mean the world to you. Start this week. Repeat every seven days.

Chapter 46

LIVE YOUR DREAM RIGHT NOW. LIVE YOUR LIFE RIGHT NOW

When you live as if your dream is already your reality, you get to test it out, see if it's all it's cracked up to be. This is also how you encourage the disparate parts of yourself to line up behind your dream, and how you quietly convince other people that you're serious about it.

People tend to argue with this suggestion. They say, "But when my dream happens, I'll be rich [famous, out of this town, married, blond, whatever]. I can't live like that now." Sure you can. What would you do if you were rich? Have nice things? Worry less about money? Live a classier life? You can do that now by disposing of any unnecessary possessions that don't seem nice and taking good care of what's left. You can get responsible about your money and replace wasteful worry with fruitful action. And you can write thank-you notes, listen to arias, and have people over for elegant little teas long before you make the *Forbes* list.

Use this process for any dream you have. What elements of it can you start living today? Doing this will help draw your dream to you and give you better odds for living it effectively. The lottery winners you hear about who blow their jackpot in a year didn't have a chance to live rich before the windfall hit. They didn't know how to sustain their newfound fortune, so it evaporated. The rueful stories of child stars, one-hit wonders, and overnight successes often share this theme: they arrived at the destination without going on the journey.

Practice may not make perfect, but it makes a great deal possible that wouldn't have been without it. Practice living your dream by imagining that you're already where you want to be. In that state, what would your day be like? What would you be like? How much of that can you put into practice now as well as later? Do it. This should be fun. If you want the life your dream brings with it, start enjoying some of its perks in previews. Maybe the person you want to be reads the *Wall Street Journal*. Why wait? You can pick one up at any newsstand. Your future self might have lots of time and money to be gracious and generous. Be gracious in the time you have and generous with the resources at your disposal. If the mother or grandmother you're hoping to be spends hours each week playing with children and helping shape their lives, become a Big Sister or a volunteer tutor. You'll be shaping some lives that are already here.

And by all means dress the part. If your dream is corporate, your suits should be too: tailored, discreet, flattering. If the dream is artistic, you get to dress like an artist—anything goes, but with style. If you want to move with the rich and powerful, you need clothing that says quality, even if the quality hung on a consignment shop hanger before getting to your closet.

If fashion intimidates you, it's probably from lack of exposure. Like enrolling in an immersion program for a foreign language, you can immerse yourself in wonderful clothes and combinations of them. Watch the makeover shows on television and peruse books about fashion at the library or bookstore. These provide the nuts and bolts. They help you find your type and zero in on what really appeals to you. Then start looking in the windows of the best shops and on the pages of the magazines. Some of the images will be outlandish, even unwearable. In those, look for individual elements that are sensational—the carved buttons maybe, or the curious juxtaposition of velvet and corduroy.

When you look in the mirror and you've dressed the part, you see an image of the person you want to be. That makes it easier to believe that this is the person you are. When other people see you in that role, their thoughts and opinions about who you are feed into the collective unconscious as well, furthering your cause in the process.

As you use your imagination to give substance to your dream, as you dress in character and live those pieces of the dream that are possible now, keep track of your progress. Do a check-in once a week, always on the same day, to see what you did this week to give your dream depth and breadth and solidity. You may even want to keep a dream log where you document the actions you took and, when appropriate, the results that came from taking them. As you get into the groove of living as if your dreams were already realized, they'll take shape more quickly. As they do, you'll have to keep up with them. In other words, when you have enough money for, say, organic produce instead of the sprayed stuff, don't stay stuck back in poor mode, regretting the cost of every carrot. Let yourself grow into your prosperity, or whatever it is you're achieving, with seamless grace.

Change is uncomfortable, even good change, but between here and the life of your dreams, you're going to have to accommodate myriad changes, the way a butterfly-in-the-making accommodates itself to one stage after another before breaking free from its cocoon. You'll do this with flawless flair by remembering the changeless part of you that came with you when you got here and will exit with you when you go. That spirit within you is the stabilizer that keeps your self-ness intact even as your dress size, your job title, your marital status, and your tax bracket go from where they are to where you want them. (This spiritual anchor is also there to sustain you should the process require that things fall apart before they come together.)

And through it all, your dual assignment is to live your dream right now, *and to live your life right now*. We have no idea the level of miracle it took to give us this chance to strut our stuff on a most obliging planet. An old story from Japan tells of a vast ocean. In the misty reaches of this nearly endless deep there is a blind sea turtle that comes to the surface only once every one hundred years. The story then asks us to imagine a small wooden ring—an embroidery hoop maybe—tossed far, far out into that titanic sea. The likelihood, the story says, that that blind sea turtle will rise to the surface through that embroidery hoop is the same likelihood as your having a life on earth. It is a rare and precious thing. You don't want to miss a minute of it—even when circumstances suggest that living your dream would require mild psychosis.

Reframe this day and get excited about it. No matter what your job is, find something cool about it and have something positive to say. A young actress I know had, for a time, a demanding and underpaid day job. When asked about it, she turned it into a humorous challenge by saying, "I work for a crazy old man in the dirtiest office you've ever seen." Another thespian who had a clerical post in a law office told people, "I baby-sit lawyers." To a large extent, your job is what you think it is. So is every other circumstance of your life. A telling passage from the Talmud puts it like this: "We don't see things the way they are. We see things the way we are."

When your attitude is elevated and your outlook upbeat, you have the prerequisite energy to dive into your day. Anytime you're thoroughly engaged in something, it can be thoroughly engaging. To that end, do whatever it takes to render "better than average" as many minutes of every day as possible. Brainstorm with your action partner about how you'll do this. Would winter mornings be lovelier if you slept on soft, flannel sheets? Would commuting be less of a drag if you got the sound system in your car fixed, or if you carpooled with somebody you really liked? Would work be more workable if you came in earlier, or switched departments, or personalized your cubicle? Would home be homier if you adopted a pair of kittens, bought flowers once a week, or sprang for a cleaning lady? Would the weekend be more wonderful if you made some plans and bought some tickets so that when the great guy does call, you get to say, "I can't this Saturday. How about next week?"

Living your dream and your life right now is not some improbable big deal like getting discovered at a soda fountain (are there still soda fountains?) or winning *America's Next Top Model*. It's simply taking the life you've got, cleaning it up a bit, and giving it a fresh coat of paint so that you'll like living in it. Then when you turn in each day at the end of it, fully cognizant that you'll never get that one back, you'll know it was worth all 1,440 minutes you invested.

Take an Action

Live your dream right now and live your life right now by doing one (or more) of the following:

1. Act, even in one small way, as if your dream were already manifest.

2. Practice living your dream by imagining what your day, your life, and you yourself will be like when it's signed, sealed, and dream-delivered.

3. Dress the part.

4. Do a weekly check-in on what you've done to bring your dream into being. Keep a dream log of the actions you've taken and the results that ensued.

5. Brainstorm with your action partner or a trusted friend about how you can upgrade various aspects of the life you have right now.

Chapter 47

YOU HAVE TO STAND FOR SOMETHING

V*alues* has become a buzzword, bantered about by politicians who speak of "our values" without asking us what they are and assuming that everyone's are the same. Despite certain values with which the majority of people in a society or community agree, values are not at their root collective. They're personal. And knowing yours will help you avoid the unpleasantness of fat, broke & lonely.

"My values spell ditch," my husband announced one evening.

"Your values spell ditch. Okay."

"Yeah: discretion, integrity, tolerance, civility, humility." It was touching. A few days before I'd gone to a workshop that dealt with defining values, and he and I had discussed the subject then. He had known his values almost immediately and now realized he could make an acronym out of them for ready recollection. His values seemed so British to me, so stiff-upper-lip, Harrow and Oxford, and yet William grew up in Liberty, Missouri. Geography notwithstanding, these truly are his values. I see in how he lives his life that "ditch" is the lodestar that guides his dealings in the world. Hearing him recite them made me fall in love all over again.

Curiously, my values—which don't spell anything that I know of—are different. Compassion is a big one. And communication. There's faith. Individuality. Irrepressibility—bouncing back from just about anything to keep on going. I don't live up to these half as much as I wish I did, but they point the way for me. And even though my list doesn't match William's, our values are compatible and so are we.

As the old adage (and not-quite-as-old country song) has it, you have to stand for something or you'll fall for anything—fat, broke & lonely, for instance. Your values are what you stand for. Some of them you got from your parents. Some are probably the opposite of your parents'. When you stay close to your values while at the same time allowing other people to have different ones, you strengthen yourself from the inside and discover gifts you didn't know were there.

What values have to do with successfully giving the boot to fat, broke & lonely is simple: having values, practicing them, and standing up for them is the surest route to owning your power. One of the recurrent negative messages that used to play in my head was, "Who do you think you are?" It was sure to crop up whenever anything incredible happened, or was about to happen, or could possibly happen. My friend Elizabeth counseled me to change the question to "Who do you *know* you are?" When I could say that I knew I was a woman who championed compassion, communication, faith, individuality, and irrepressibility, I was no longer just one more girl from Kansas City making her way as best she could. I was a woman of substance with work to do and a reason to be here.

This is how I see it: on your own, you're a person trying to get by like everybody else. With your values, you take on the strength of conviction and the legacy of everyone who's gone before you who also carried the banner for nonviolence or equality or rights for somebody who doesn't have enough of them. Having values doesn't alter your personal worth, because your worth is inherent in your being. Your perception of that worth, however, can change tremendously. In addition, having values takes the focus off the little self and shifts it to the bigger picture.

Where this can get tricky is when we believe that our values are the only ones worth having and that anyone with other values must be wrong. It's a delicate balance to stay true to your convictions, whatever the cost, and yet give others the same right.

This is without question a sophisticated concept. It's hard enough to climb from "gimme-gimme," the ego's basic position, to espousing values that ask us to turn from that to something higher. To go on from there and willingly allow other people to live in different ways, espouse different moral precepts, and even worship a (seemingly) different God is huge. It calls for sophisticated thinking, the ability to wholeheartedly believe in something and yet keep the door open to discussion and forbearance and the possibility that in the vastness of the universe, both ways could be right. Or perhaps that being right was never the issue at all.

It's natural to want definitive answers, but sometimes there aren't any. When that's the case, the surest route to take is to love as best you can, live as fully as possible, and turn in your curly white wig because judging everybody else doesn't change anything for the better. Maybe not everyone is required to live and let live in this way. Somebody you know may be able to be rigid and holier-than-us and a totally pompous ass and do just fine. But if you want to call it quits with fat, broke & lonely, you have a different path to walk. That path calls for having values that give you purpose, living them as well as you're able, and giving other people the freedom to do the same.

Take an Action

Pick one of your values and focus on living it today with all your heart. Tonight look back on how that went. Do you feel any stronger than usual? Were you able to live your value without denying your fellow people the right to live theirs?

Chapter 48

KEEP ADDING TO
THE SOUP

Soup is the most versatile of dishes. It can be an appetizer or an entrée, chunky or pureed, steaming or chilled. You can thin it or thicken it, accommodate a crowd with a few more carrots and potatoes and peas, even transform Monday's soup into Tuesday's stew. This penchant for refurbishment makes soup a lot like us—people committed to hooking up with the life of our dreams and living, if not *happily* ever after, *fully* ever after and happy much of the time.

"Keep adding to the soup" is a humble kitchen metaphor for enriching your life with color and texture, substance and spice. It doesn't just give you permission to explore new ideas and different ways of looking at things; it says that if you don't, your life forever after will be cream of tomato, cream of tomato, cream of tomato—and from a can at that.

To rescue you from this no-cook's-land, here are some specifics you may wish to add to the pot:

- *Keep learning all the time.* Keep learning even when you're out of school, reading with bifocals, and getting the senior discount for lectures at the Y. One common theme in many of the reports of people who have allegedly had near-death experiences is that they were asked two questions: "Did you learn how to love?" "What else did you learn?" So for the joy of your life (and, gosh, maybe your afterlife), learn stuff! Learn about things and learn to do things. What interests you? What did you avoid studying in school because it was too hard or too easy or not in your focus area? Take the class now. Read the book. Rent the documentary.

- *Stir in some travel.* Getting places is faster and cheaper than earlier generations could have imagined, and despite security checks and the prudent need to avoid some places in the world for now, travel is still transformative. Until you've put your foot on the other side of the globe, you don't really know it's there. Once you have, you become a planetary citizen, and nothing that happens anywhere is ever again fully divorced from your own life.

- *Get to know people.* Talk to strangers. Ask children what they think of things and ask old people about their lives. Find out what it was like to grow up in Newcastle or New Delhi, what a Mormon or a Mennonite believes, how the world looks to an Icelander or an Iowan.

- *Mix it up.* You have the right to try out different jobs, different locations, and different ways of being in the world. The sabbatical so prized in academic circles is a tradition that needs to be expanded far and wide. If you don't have a year to explore something that has long fascinated you, take a week or an hour or whatever you've got.

- *Store beautiful images.* Take pictures, with your camera or with your brain, of everything you come across that is particularly beautiful. It may be a panorama of the forest or one crimson leaf, the face of your lover or your toddler smeared with jam and smiling. Look for these. Listen for them. Go out of your way to find them, and when you do, give them a bit of your time. Make the little things—the fruit bowl on your table, the floor of your closet, your desk when you leave for the evening—as beautiful as they can be in a real-world real life where fruit gets eaten, shoes get tossed, and papers proliferate.

- *Gather words of wisdom and wonder.* This is alphabet soup with a purpose. The ingredients are words, phrases, quotations, lines of poetry, slabs of Shakespeare. Write them down. Memorize the best ones. These words and the ideas they carry will be companions and instructors for you. Sometimes when you're in the throes of a dilemma, Lao-tzu or Sojourner Truth or Ethel Merman will have the answer. When you can pull it from your memory bank, your journal, or your hard drive, you have the answer too.

- *Fill up your senses.* Your body needs sweet good things as much as your mind and soul do. It wants to walk in the rain and jump in puddles (rubber boots are a wondrous invention). It wants to hike in the mud and smell October and taste snow. It's yearning right now for a long bath or a back rub, a warmer coat or darker sunglasses. Listen to it and give it a plethora of delights.

- *Fill in the missing parts.* It's important to know who you are and to be who are, to spend time on what lights you up and with the people who make you feel welcome and appreciated. Even so, you are a multifaceted being, and some of those facets you haven't discovered yet. Therefore, if you're a city girl, go camping. If you never knew your grandparents, volunteer at a nursing home. If you live in your head, do something with your hands. Not every foray into unfamiliar territory will yield something of lasting value, but each step in that direction is an experience for the record and might just get you closer to your dream.

- *Don't miss out.* Or as Emerson put it: "Do not be too timid and squeamish about your actions. All life is an experience." So experience it! Of course do what you have to do, and what you have to do may at times require self-sacrifice and putting off your desires for the time being for some greater good. But the over-whelming majority of the time, if you really want to do something, find a way. Otherwise, your life ends up beige and gray with maybe a daring splash of khaki. That may be a step up from fat, broke & lonely, but not much of one. If you're willing to put forth the effort, reschedule the commitments, or rearrange the budget so that you can have it, do it, or go there—you deserve the joy and the memory.

The essence of adding to the soup is to continually make your life richer. The more experiences you chalk up, the more tantalizing your life becomes, until one day you discover it's the one you've wanted from as far back as you can remember.

Take an Action

Add to the soup today some pungent pastime, savory skill, or exotic experience of your choosing.

Chapter 49

WHEN YOU DON'T WANT TO DO THIS STUFF, YOU NEED IT MORE THAN EVER

When you're feeling on top of the world—confident, competent, attractive, and energized—there's nothing you can't do. Other times it can seem impossible to put forth effort, even to take care of yourself. This might happen when you're out of your element, perhaps in a job or location that makes you feel as if a piece of yourself was left behind and should arrive one of these days via parcel post. Or it could be that the part of you that doesn't believe you deserve the best has convinced every other part to test that hypothesis. Or maybe you're just going through a down time. Lethargy, disinterest, and residing in the dumps for more than a day or so put up a big detour sign that tells the life of your dreams to head the other way.

If you even think you may be dealing with clinical depression or highs and lows that are higher and lower than those of the people around you, you need more targeted help than can come in a book. If you're just experiencing garden-variety blahs, however, you can call their bluff by treating yourself so well that they have no choice but to take their gloom and doom elsewhere. The same goes for anytime you'd rather be court-martialed than make your bed (or even get out of it). *When you don't want to do this stuff, you need it more than ever.* This includes everything you've been reading about: meditation, exercise, eating healthy food in reasonable quantities, earning enough to avoid stress and using the money you have wisely, enjoying alone time, meeting new people and keeping in touch with the ones already in your life, and staying focused on your dream.

On days when you look at that list and it reads like "climb Kilimanjaro, cure cancer, and discover a new planet," come up with *minimums* that you're committed to doing on good days and bad, no matter what. To figure out your minimums, look at fat, broke & lonely. Determine which of these has been your biggest problem and is most likely to come up from behind and cause you trouble. Based on this, your minimums—the steps you take every day, so help you God— might be getting some exercise, being sure to eat a salad, and checking in with your action partner. Someone else's minimums might be washing her hair and wearing makeup, writing down the money she spends, and taking one action toward looking for a better job. You determine your minimums because you know your life.

This is not to say that you're supposed to hide behind your minimums forever ("I never have to exercise; I'm only dealing with money issues"). But on days when doing anything at all seems like a monumental undertaking, your minimums are the few things you'll absolutely do, no matter how overwhelming the rest of it seems. Here are some additional ideas that should help:

- *Buy a kind clock.* Getting started is key. Whether you're a cheerful morning person or the pre-noon hours offend your sensibilities, treat yourself to a clock that doesn't shock the bejesus out of you. There are clocks that awaken you with the gentle chimes of a Zen monastery, or that slowly light up the room, or that let you awaken to your favorite music or even a prerecorded wake-up message you made just for yourself.

- *Decide your mood for the day while you're still in bed.* If you wait to find out that it's raining, your hair is frizzy, and you managed to grow a pimple the size of Delaware overnight, these circumstances beyond your control could shape your outlook. Don't give them the chance. Acknowledge before your feet touch the floor that you're damn lucky to have this day, no matter what it (or you) looks like.

- *Find the little things that get you through.* Some days you do everything required of you just because it's required of you. Other days you need help. For example, let's say you have to get to work super-early. If you have your coffee at home, you might never want to leave. If instead you plan to buy coffee en route, you've got yourself a cupful of motivation.

- *This time, don't be creative.* When your mood is puny at best, don't think of interesting alternative ways to conduct yourself. Believe me, they won't be interesting. On a day like this, go through the motions you've established and accomplish your minimums, or a little bit more. Get up. Wash face. Use deodorant. Do ten minutes of easy yoga. Feed fish. Feed self. Dress. Play happy CD in car. Get to office and actually say, "Good morning" (by now you might almost believe it is a good morning).

- *Just get out.* On schloggy days, you sometimes just need to get the momentum going. You do this by getting out. Go out for breakfast, go out to the gym, go out to run errands—it doesn't matter so much what you do as that you get your body out into the world. Putting yourself into the flow of life can convince you that you actually want to be there.

- *Break up tasks into reasonable pieces.* Otherwise, you may feel overwhelmed by all there is to do. Try looking separately at the obligations in the various areas of your life. Having all your work duties, home chores, spouse-and-kids stuff, and organizational and volunteer tasks on one to-do list might be appropriate for an upbeat, high-energy day, but when you're not a reasonable replica of Little Mary Sunshine, it could be debilitating.

- *Aptly employ both inspiration and distraction.* Inspiration—whether from reading something encouraging, watching a show about someone who overcame the odds, or looking through the latest Pottery Barn catalog to remind yourself how pretty life can be—works wonders when you're feeling glum, even if you write off this kind of thing as cloying the rest of the time. In addition, carefully applied distraction has its place. Try raucous music to distract you while you're cleaning house. Listen to a friend's agonies (or ecstasies) to distract you from your own. Tune in to an hour of escapist TV to distract you from reality as we know it.

- *Focus on the other people in your life.* When you don't want to take care of yourself, chances are you're not thrilled about taking care of other people either, and yet it's sometimes easier to get back on course by rousing yourself to do something for someone else.

- *Take a personal day once in a while.* And because it's personal, you can do with it whatever you like, such as lazing around and thinking about how dumb your dream is and deciding that if you can avoid fat, broke & lonely by just a hair, you don't need any more than that. Fine. But remember: it's a personal *day*, not a personal decade.

Because life is cyclical and we are too, there will be times when your energy lags and your resolve is less than steely. During these periods, just stay above the break-even point. Do what you need to do, if only just your minimums, so you know you aren't losing ground. After you've done that much, it feels good to think you've earned the enjoyment that follows. When the workday is over and the house is clean and you want to go out for dinner with friends or stay in and watch HBO, you can know that whatever you feel like doing with your evening is your just desserts.

Take an Action

Figure out for yourself what your minimums are. What has to happen just about every day for you to feel that you're at least breaking even? Be realistic and make these your absolute minimums. Remember, this is what you intend to accomplish on those days when you really don't want to accomplish anything.

Chapter 50

IF YOU KNEW WHO YOU REALLY WERE, YOU'D BE STARSTRUCK

There may have been great whopping millennia when just getting by was fine. You don't happen to be living in one of those. You've got yourself a life smack inside the Chinese double entendre "May you live in interesting times." Not to be overly dramatic, but you have a responsibility to pull out every seed of wisdom, courage, and potential inside yourself, plant it, water it, and harvest it. Personal growth—striving for what psychologist Abraham Maslow labeled "self-actualization"—has always called for this. Our "interesting times" demand it.

If you were to stick a pin in every point on a tabletop globe where there is danger or unease or an incipient threat, it would look like a spherical porcupine. What do you think would happen to all that unease and unrest if each one of us tapped into who we really are? If everybody on earth did this, there would be a change like the world has never seen. The French scientist and theologian Pierre Teilhard de Chardin predicted something like this when he wrote, "The day will come when, after harnessing space, the winds, the tides, gravitation, we shall harness for God the energies of love. And on that day, for the second time in the history of the world, man will have discovered fire."

But what if only a smattering of us, the people who read this book, were to do it? Even if the relative few of us who are finished with fat, broke & lonely were to fathom our true identity and commit ourselves to living up to the highest light that's in us, we could bring forth a gentle revolution, a surge of change. You see, there's a point to kicking fat, broke & lonely to the curb that goes beyond the satisfaction of the act and the pleasure of your freedom: once you're free, you're free to be remarkable.

You have the right stuff already. It's factory-installed. The Gandhis, Mother Teresas, and Martin Luther Kings of this world aren't qualitatively different from the rest of us. They just go deeper within themselves. They're scared like we are, but they keep on marching. No matter how many people tell them to be practical or to grow up and deal with things the way they are, they have the chutzpah to be impractical and to change the way things are. You can join them. It is, in fact, your obligation to join them.

You are fully capable. You may want to acquire more facts or gain more experience (and be absolutely certain you're out of the woods with fat, broke & lonely) before you take on the contemporary equivalent of Jim Crow or the British empire. Nevertheless, you are capable today of having on the world an impact for good. Maybe today you'll only write a letter to an editor or pick up groceries for an elderly neighbor, but the ripple effect of such actions cancels out the "only."

It's a great shock when you reach adulthood to realize that all those grown-ups you'd thought were on top of everything don't know any more than you do. Even the professors and the presidents are piecing it together as best they can. Here's your job: piece it together better. Do that by tapping into the highest and best that's in you, even when your self-interest would rather see you doing something else.

It is true that to get over fat, broke & lonely you have to humble yourself and see that you're not the center of the universe. It is equally true that to go on to live a remarkable life you have to acknowledge the immeasurable power inside you that can be put to good purpose. *If you knew who you really were, you'd be starstruck.* Not only are there atoms in your body that were in dinosaurs and Moses and Marilyn Monroe, but you have a direct line to greatness. Your bright ideas ("Where'd that come from?") and your right-on hunches ("How did I know that?") are drawn from the same well of genius as Einstein's and Beethoven's. If they had brushed off their excellence, we wouldn't have heard of them either.

Everybody has access to what I think of as divine ideas. I'm biased toward *your* access to them because I know, as someone who has also faced fat, broke & lonely, how dealing with that kind of darkness can make you so ready to let in some light. It's not just food and money and aloneness that can put somebody in this state: any kind of addiction will do it, or a serious illness, or a heavy loss. Whatever gets you there, coming out on the other side lets you glimpse what was in you all along: more power and light than you could get from a good-sized utility company. Curiously, the very thing that may have made you feel most ashamed, most unsuited to doing anything spectacular, becomes the portal into the life you were meant for all along.

Until you realize this—and renew the realization as needed—it's easy to feel like a nobody. It's a big world. You spend a lot of your life working your way up and dealing with people above you who seem to have taken weekend seminars in how to make you feel small. It doesn't matter if you're the person who makes the coffee instead of the decisions: don't let anybody fool you into thinking you're nothing. In that state, you can't access your brilliance. But you need your brilliance. So do all the rest of us.

Sure, adversity will show its ugly mug. You're not going to read this book and be forever immune to the lure of the wrong kind of guy or the right kind of bakery, but you'll recognize what's happening and change course. And even if you don't always change course right away—good Lord, we're human—you won't spend months beating yourself up for not being perfect. You'll use mistakes for making your own wisdom, the way your body uses sunlight on your skin to make vitamin D. And you'll start to learn a whole lot faster. You won't make the same kinds of mistakes over and over. You can be imperfect in all sorts of interesting ways—far better to have well-rounded imperfections than the stuck-in-a-rut kind.

As you progress toward your dream, there will be obstacles. If the process were easy, it wouldn't be a dream, just the next notation on your to-do list that you could check off before lunchtime. A dream or a goal is by nature fraught with peril. You have to be confident that even if you despair briefly in the face of apparent failure, you'll regroup and go forward.

Everything that's happened to you so far is part of your journey. You have the option now to steer the journey's course. You've decided to split for good with fat, broke & lonely. The upshot of that decision is that you'll take whatever action is necessary whenever it is necessary to live sanely and serenely, even if you'd rather eat another cupcake or buy some tantalizing electronic gizmo with the rent money. To live sanely and serenely, you have a Higher Power and your inner power, which is basically the Higher Power filtered through you. With all that going for you, you can live a remarkable life. And you can make a remarkable difference.

Take an Action

Just sit—sometime today, or tomorrow morning when you have your quiet time—with the notion that you have the power within you to live a remarkable life. It's nothing to get cocky about—after all, you didn't put it there—but it is essential that you recognize it. You have every right to live free from fat, broke & lonely. You also have a responsibility to live your best life. I'd thought about calling this chapter "Who Am I Supposed to Be, Mahatma Gandhi?" The answer would have been, well, sort of. You're supposed to be yourself certainly, but also a *mahatma,* a "great soul." It's in you already. Your action to take, every day of your life, is to live like you know that.

ACKNOWLEDGMENTS

I am in awe of authors whose acknowledgments run to one tasteful paragraph thanking their agent, editor, and significant other. For me, every book is a collaboration, and I love naming the people who contributed.

Like those authors with less-is-more acknowledgments, I'll start with my agent, and my friend, Linda Chester. If I tell all the ways she's wonderful, other writers will come after me and demand to know how I got so lucky. I don't know how. I only know that I'm grateful every day to have an agent who believes so deeply in what I do and exhibits nonstop generosity, intelligence, graciousness, and loyalty.

Next come all the terrific people at HarperOne and HarperCollins, particularly my editor, Gideon Weil, who was the first to see "fat, broke & lonely" as an issue to address. Thanks for your skill and hard work, and for having me as part of the HarperCollins family.

As for significant others, my dear husband, William Melton, has provided unflagging support and unwavering understanding. He thinks I'm remarkable, and that makes me want to be. My lovely daughter, Adair Moran, brainstormed with me over many a latté and encouraged me immensely when she said early on: "I know this is a book you can write." Thank you for your help on this book and your patience through all of them.

Thanks to my talented assistant, Joya Scott, who, in handling with efficiency and ease everything I used to trip over, enabled me to focus on writing. Thanks also to Gary Jaffe, Linda Chester's unflappable assistant, attorney Dennis Dahlrymple, and Whitney Lee, my foreign rights agent, who'll take this book into the wider world.

My action partner, Sherry Boone, has been almost a co-author, inspiring me throughout and sharing selflessly of her own experience and wisdom. Olivia Fox of Spitfire Communications has been equally instrumental as an ongoing mentor and invaluable resource. Special thanks to Alima for her guidance at the outset of this project and support throughout. Thanks also to Crystal Leaman, who helped me clarify my message and remember my purpose in writing this book; to my vision partner, Randy Ladner; and to the Rev. Paul Tenaglia and the Rev. Chris Michaels for holding this vision so steadily that I had to come through. And to my wonderful life-coaching clients: I work for you, but you do so much for me.

Thanks to the New York City focus group—Hsin-Cha Hsu, Dr. Lorna Flamer-Caldera, Alice Marie, Nava Namdar, and Sarah Williams—who got me focused early in the project. Others whose suggestions and encouragement nestle within these pages include Laura Allen, Hilda Bennett, Barbara Biziou, Patti Breitman, Dr. T. Colin Campbell, Dr. Pauline

Canelias, Rosemary Cathcart, Susan Cheever, Elizabeth Cutting, Necia Gamby, John Taylor Gatto, Jan Goldstoff, Amy Gonigam, Dominque Guerin, Donna Henes, Sharmaine Hobbs, the Rev. Evan Howard, Kevin Kelly, Jodi Leib, Leslie Levine, Sasha Lodi, Betty Melton, Siân Melton, Cathryn Michon, Nicholas A. Moran, Jerry Mundis, Alysia Reiner, Linda Ruocco, Thom Rutledge, Carol Shiflett, Deborah Shouse, Wendy Spero, Carol Stillman, Letitia Suk, Heather Traber-Fitzgerald, and Jamie Zaffos, as well as the late Dr. Richard Carlson who taught me to write early in the morning, keep chapters short and concepts accessible, and of course, not sweat the small stuff.

To the cherished friends and family members—you know who you are—who kept this book in your prayers during its lengthy birthing process, you're in my prayers now. To Ann Estrada and the rest of the staff at the neighborhood Starbucks where I wrote a great deal of both this book and my previous one: you're the best. And to Karen Morella and the Serendipity B&B in Ocean City, New Jersey, where I retreated for literary inspiration: it worked, and your scrambled tofu is out of this world.

Heartfelt thanks to the Saturday morning writers' group that kept me going, the 7:15 A.M. meetings that kept me centered, and Unity of New York City, where weekly infusions of energy and uplift fueled *Fat, Broke & Lonely No More* into being.

Finally, I wish to thank you, the reader, for giving this book your time and attention. Nothing would please me more than to know that it spoke to you and helped you live a grander life. Based on readership of my previous works and the "standard profile" of readers of books like this, there's a 94 percent likelihood that you're a woman (for books with pink covers, it's probably 98 percent). To those men who are reading this anyway (especially those who have written me over the years to say, "We are out here and we read too"), I see you guys as the few, the proud, the gutsy. Although I have written largely to the majority, I have kept you gentlemen in mind and made non-gender-specific comments whenever I could. When I typed "bikini waxing" in chapter 44, I thought, "Oh, my gosh. Men will cringe." But you obviously handled it just fine.

BIBLIOGRAPHY

The books listed here include those alluded to in *Fat, Broke &
Lonely No More* as well as others—some recent, some clas-
sics in their field—that I believe can help you keep fat, broke
& lonely in the past and live a remarkable life. This is by no
means an exhaustive list, but every book here is one that I've
read all the way through and thoroughly stand behind.

Bailey, Covert. *The New Fit or Fat.* Boston: Houghton Mifflin,
1991. Since their inception in the 1970s, the *Fit or Fat* books
and philosophy have explained what's *really* the problem with
fat and shown how the right kind of exercise can help solve
it. Bailey has retired, but there's information about his work
on the website of his colleague Ronda Gates, www.ronda-
gates.com.

Beak, Sera. *The Red Book: A Deliciously Unorthodox Approach to Ig-
niting Your Inner Spark.* Hoboken, N.J.: Jossey-Bass, 2006 (www.
serabeak.com). This is a wondrously revolutionary book

about spirituality for women in their twenties. The author is herself a savvy, stylish young woman who holds a master's degree in theology from Harvard and has whirled with dervishes in Turkey, volunteered at Mother Teresa's Home for the Dying in Calcutta, and had an audience with the Dalai Lama on her twenty-first birthday.

Beherndt, Greg, and Liz Tuccillo. *He's Just Not That into You: The No-Excuses Truth to Understanding Guys.* New York: Simon Spotlight Entertainment, 2004. In this best-seller, two former writers for *Sex and the City* help women give up on lost-cause relationships and find a man who really cares.

Berthold-Bond, Annie. *Clean and Green: The Complete Guide to Nontoxic and Environmentally Safe Housekeeping.* Woodstock, N.Y.: Ceres Press, 1994 (www.betterbasics.com). I mentioned this book in the chapter "Put Your Money Where Your Morals Are." I've been using its housecleaning recipes for years and I hate tidying up somewhat less than before I got creative about it.

Bolen, Jean Shinoda, M.D. *The Millionth Circle: How to Change Ourselves and the World—The Essential Guide to Women's Circles.* Newburyport, Mass.: Conari Press, 1999 (www.jeanbolen. com). If you want to gather with women to make a difference for yourself and the world, this little book has all you need to know.

Campbell, T. Colin, and Thomas M. Campbell II. *The China Study: The Most Comprehensive Study of Nutrition Ever Conducted & the Startling Implications for Diet, Weight Loss, and Long-Term Health.* Dallas: Benbella Books, 2006. (www.thechinastudy.com). The results of the nuturitional study the *New York Times* called "the Grand Prix of epidemiology." Conclusion: a whole foods, largely vegetarian diet is your best bet for a lean body and healthy life.

Chambers, Veronica. *The Joy of Doing Things Badly: A Girl's Guide to Love, Life, and Foolish Bravery.* New York: Broadway Books, 2006 (www.veronicachambers.com). With perfection promulgated far and wide, Chambers suggests that a willingness to fall flat heightens life's joys. A girlfriend-to-girlfriend book weighing in on work, friendship, success, failure, and what the author learned from Julia Child.

Cheever, Susan. *American Bloomsbury: Louisa May Alcott, Ralph Waldo Emerson, Margaret Fuller, Nathaniel Hawthorne, and Henry David Thoreau: Their Lives, Their Loves, Their Work.* New York: Simon & Schuster, 2006. Provides juicy background information on Emerson and his amazing colleagues.

Chopra, Deepak, M.D. *Perfect Health: The Complete Mind/Body Guide.* New York: Three Rivers Press, 1991, 2000 (www.chopra.com). I read this book over and over. Doing what it says helps me stay healthy and eat and live in a way that's full of ease and satisfaction.

Critser, Greg. *Fat Land: How Americans Became the Fattest People in the World.* Boston: Houghton Mifflin/Mariner, 2003. An absorbing journalistic exposé of the factors leading to the obesity epidemic.

Daddona, Cynthia. *Diary of a Modern-Day Goddess.* Deerfield Beach, Fla.: HCI, 2000 (www.moderndaygoddess.com). A lovely, lighthearted guide to taking exquisite care of yourself, body and soul. Daddona's "A Balanced Modern-Day Goddess To-Do List for the Month" is worth the price of the book.

Dennis, Patrick. *Auntie Mame: An Irreverent Escapade*. New York: Broadway Books, 2001. This is the charming 1956 tale that inspired the film I recommended in "Fill Your Life, Then Your Plate." If you're looking for a mentor on living well, Mame's your gal.

Dominguez, Joe, and Vicki Robins. *Your Money or Your Life: Transforming Your Relationship with Money and Achieving Financial Independence*, rev. ed. New York: Penguin, 1999 (www.newroad-map.org). This was the first book to enlighten me to the fact that money and life aren't meant to be at odds, that financial freedom is indeed possible, and that financial independence and being a good planetary citizen are compatible after all.

Dunnan, Nancy. *How to Invest $50 to $5,000: The Small Investor's Step-by Step, Dollar-by-Dollar Plan for Low-Risk, High-Value Investing*. New York: HarperCollins, 2003 (www.nancydunnan.com). A totally non-intimidating guide for the novice (or nervous) investor.

Emerson, Ralph Waldo. *Essays* (1926). New York: Harper-Perennial, (www.transcendentalists.com). "The Over-Soul" is a wonderful look at the concept of God for those at odds with traditional definitions, and essays on "Prudence" and "Friendship" offer wise insights into broke and lonely.

Friends of Peace Pilgrim. *Peace Pilgrim: Her Life and Work in Her Own Words*. Santa Fe, N.M.: Ocean Tree, 1992 (www.peace-pilgrim.com). Peace Pilgrim was a modern mystic who said things like, "Live up to the highest light you have and more light will be given to you." I reread this book periodically, as well as the 365-entry daybook *Peace Pilgrim's Wisdom: A Very Simple Guide*, edited by Cheryl Canfield (Santa Fe, N.M.: Ocean Tree, 1996).

Gatto, John Taylor. *Dumbing Us Down: The Hidden Curriculum of Compulsory Schooling*. Gabriola Island, B.C.: New Society Publishers, 2005. The book that introduced me to the fascinating views of this maverick educator, onetime New York state Teacher of the Year, whose ideas I allude to in Chapter 3.

Grout, Pam. *God Doesn't Have Bad Hair Days: Ten Spiritual Experiments That Will Bring More Abundance, Joy, and Love to Your Life*. Philadelphia: Running Press, 2005 (www.pamgrout.com). Grout asks readers to test out the God theory with experiments like "Godlets R Us" and "The Sally Field Principle: The Dude Likes You. He Really Likes You."

Hay, Louise L. *I Can Do It! How to Use Affirmations to Change Your Life*. Carlsbad, Calif.: Hay House, 2004 (www.louisehay.com). Affirmations have been around long enough that it's easy to say, "Oh yeah, *those*." *I Can Do It*, from the woman who is largely responsible for putting affirmations on the map in the first place, is a fresh new take on this useful tool as a way to attract love and romance, self-esteem, a new job, and all sorts of good stuff. The book comes with a CD and has spawned calendars and other goodies.

Houston, Jean, Ph.D. *A Passion for the Possible: A Guide to Realizing Your True Potential*. San Francisco: HarperSanFrancisco, 1998 (www.jeanhouston.org). A guide to understanding the four levels of self—sensory/physical, psychological, mythic/symbolic, and spiritual—through exercise and meditation. The bagel-eating and show tune–listening that Houston inspired in me is part of why, when I look up from my computer, I have a view of the Chrysler Building.

Ilibagiza, Immaculee. *Left to Tell: Finding God Amidst the Rwandan Holocaust.* Carlsbad, Calif.: Hay House, 2005 (www.lefttotell.com). This is not a self-help book; it is a self-healing book—and a planetary-healing book besides. The author made her way through unimaginable horrors through the power of forgiveness. I assign *Left to Tell* to many of my coaching clients. No one has ever said that it failed to change her life.

Kramer, Sarah, and Tanya Barnard. *How It All Vegan: Irresistible Recipes for an Animal-Free Diet.* Vancouver, B.C.: Arsenal Pulp Press, 2001 (www.govegan.net). More than a cookbook (it even has beauty tips), this fresh, sassy guide with a post-punk sensibility was written by two young proponents of green cuisine and is filled with both yummy recipes and cheeky style. Its sequel, *The Garden of Vegan: How It All Vegan Again* (Vancouver, B.C.: Arsenal Pulp Press, 2003), carries the tradition forward.

Krishnamurti, J. *At the Feet of the Master.* Wheaton, Ill.: Theosophical Publishing House, 1994. A tiny classic from the very young Krishnamurti and the source of the quotation about your body being the "horse upon which you ride." For more on Krishnamurti and his later teachings, see the Krishnamurti Foundation of America website, www.kfa.org.

Michaels, Chris. *Your Soul's Assignment*. Kansas City, Mo.: Awakening World Enterprises, 2003 (www.yoursoulsassignment.com). Chris Michaels is one of my spiritual teachers, and this book gives you his no-holds-barred take on what you're here for.

Michon, Cathryn. *The Grrl Genius Guide to Sex (with Other People): A Self-Help Novel*. New York: St. Martin's Press, 2004 (www.grrlgenius.com). Relationship lessons from one who's been in the trenches and stuck it out with humor (Michon is a stand-up comic and comedy writer) to a *very* happy ending. This "self-help novel" features tips in boxes and charts (for example, "Drawbacks to Being Beautiful"). Michon's first book, *The Grrl Genius Guide to Life: A Twelve-Step Program on How to Become a Grrl Genius, According to Me!* (New York: HarperCollins, 2001), is another winner.

Moran, Victoria. *Creating a Charmed Life: Sensible, Spiritual Secrets Every Busy Woman Should Know*. San Francisco: HarperSan-Francisco, 1999 (www.victoriamoran.com). Once you're over fat, broke & lonely, you may as well live a charmed life. The seventy-five bite-sized essays in this book will teach you everything from how to play your free square (like in Bingo, but this one's in life) to how to practice the vacation principle so you live like you're on vacation every day.

———. *Fit from Within: 101 Simple Secrets to Change Your Body and Your Life*. New York: Contemporary Books/McGraw-Hill, 2003; audiobook, Toronto: SimplyAudio (www.simplyaudio.com), 2006. I don't mean to be greedy in recommending two of my own books, but I honestly believe they both could help you. This one goes into detail about how you can lose extra weight and keep it off indefinitely without deprivation or re-incarnating in another body.

Mundis, Jerrold. *How to Get Out of Debt, Stay Out of Debt, and Live Prosperously*. New York: Bantam, 1988 (www.mundismoney. com). I think I'm safe in saying that if I'd never read this book, I'd probably still be broke. Based on the proven principles and techniques of Debtors Anonymous, this one is a keeper.

Newkirk, Ingrid. *The Compassionate Cook: Please Don't Eat the Animals*. New York: Warner Books, 1993 (www.goveg.com). Easy, animal-free recipes from the founder of PETA. I use this cookbook all the time.

Rippe, David, and Jared Rosen. *The Flip: Turn Your World Around!* Charlottesville, Va.: Hampton Roads Publishing, 2006 (www. theflip.net). A book about turning around the upside-down world of fear and competition to see a right-side-up world in areas including health, diet, relationships, and world affairs. Contains practical suggestions called "flip tips" and lots of fascinating stats, like those three thousand marketing mes-sages we're exposed to every day.

Rutledge, Thom. *Embracing Fear and Finding the Courage to Live Your Life*. San Francisco: HarperSanFrancisco, 2002 (www. thomrutledge.com). Psychotherapist Rutledge suggests deal-ing with fear by facing, exploring, accepting, and responding to it, thereby releasing its grip.

Schaefer, Jenni, with Thom Rutledge. *Life Without Ed: How One Woman Declared Independence from Her Eating Disorder and How You*

Can Too. New York: McGraw-Hill, 2004 (www.jennischaefer. com). One woman's story and an extremely helpful guide if your relationship with fat has sent you in the direction of anorexia, bulimia, compulsive dieting, or excessive exercise.

Shinn, Florence Scovel. *The Game of Life and How to Play It.* Marina del Rey, Calif.: DeVorss & Co., 1925 (www.florence-scovelshinn.com). It's labeled "a prosperity classic," but it's really a metaphysical classic: practical, useful, and, despite quaint references from its era, as relevant today as it was in 1925. If you love this book as I do, you'll want to get *The Writings of Florence Scovel Shinn* (also from DeVorss), which includes all Shinn's writings.

Smith, Huston. *The Religions of Man.* San Francisco: Harper-SanFrancisco, 1991 (www.hustonsmith.net). This is the only book I was assigned in college that I still read and cherish. Although spirituality and religion can be intimately related or light-years apart, I find that familiarity with the basic tenets of the major religions helps fill in some blank spots in my own spirituality. At this point in history, I also believe it's essential that we have at least a rudimentary understanding of how other people see life and faith; this book provides that clearly and with a passion that's contagious.

Spero, Wendy. *Microthrills: True Stories from a Life of Small Highs.* New York: Hudson Street Press, 2006 (www.wendyspero.com). You think you had it bad? At least your mom wasn't a sex therapist who'd walk in on you and your boyfriend and tell you just keep on going. Wendy Spero is a young comedian, and her reading for the audio version of this memoir will have you in stitches.

Stahl, Louann. *A Most Surprising Song: Exploring the Mystical Experience.* Unity Village, Mo.: Unity Books, 1992. An easy-to-read explanation of the mystical experience and some of the fascinating people who have had one. I reread this book periodically and refer to it often. It is inexplicably out of print, but you can find it in libraries and from purveyors of used books, both actual and online.

Stanny, Barbara. *Overcoming Underearning: Overcome Your Money Fears and Earn What You Deserve.* New York: HarperCollins, 2005 (www.barbarastanny.com). Clearly explaining the often self-imposed state of underearning, Stanny spells out five steps to financial freedom: tell the truth, make a decision, stretch, create community, and respect and appreciate money.

Walters, J. Donald. *Money Magnetism: How to Attract What You Need When You Need It.* Nevada City, Calif.: Crystal Clarity Publishers, 2000. This is the book I was reading when the guy in the subway handed me a dollar and said, "This stuff really works."

Zukav, Gary. *The Seat of the Soul.* New York: Fireside, 1990 (www.zukav.com). An eclectic guide to serious spirituality that includes chapters on addiction and relationships.

To contact the author, subscribe to her free ezine "The Charmed Monday Minute," inquire about life-coaching services, or book her to speak for your organization, visit her website: www.victoriamoran.com.